POETIC SYMBIOSIS III

Poetic Symbiosis Three

Embracing Addiction and Mental Illness

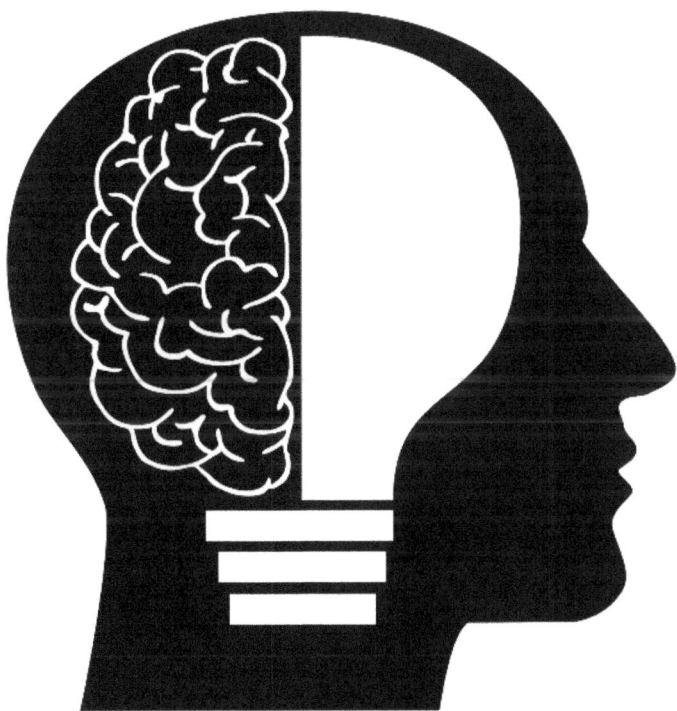

Matt Loat and Docrobin

This edition published 2022 by:

Takahe Publishing Ltd.

Registered Office:

77 Earlsdon Street, Coventry CV5 6EL

ISBN 978-1-908837-24-0

TAKAHE PUBLISHING LTD.

2022

This final volume in the trilogy is dedicated once more to the lasting memory of Allan Peter Toft and Mark Vincent Loat. Also to Marie May (notre bête noire). Yet again, it spurred us on to continue our efforts in illustrating such complex issues for our readers, using both our own experiences and those of others we have encountered in our own journeys.

Acknowledgements

We would like to thank the following for their continued support, understanding and friendship as part of our extended networks:

Yvonne, Samantha, Amber, Duncan, Diane, Lee, Fern, Harvey, Leo, Russell, Chris, Mikayla, Shannan, Jenna, Emily S, Benjamin, Mary, Anita, Hazel, Adrian, Sarah, Benita, Mark W, Terry, Agro, Mark L, Madison, Noah, KT, Harper, David C, Amanda B, Xander C, Kai C, Iain C, Kayleigh C, Emma S, Duane H, Lexi L, Oscar L, Anna B, Simon P, Kam S, Patricia C, Bob R, Ian F, Carole D (Dec'd), Marie M, Prince M, Emily T, Rednits, Anne B, Colin S, Emilie LJ, Steve H

CONTENTS

Part II: A Rational Approach to Therapeutic Support (RATS)?

Introduction

Blimey! Matt and the Doc strike again with a third volume about mental health and addiction! They have produced an awful lot of material over the past couple of years, in spite of a pandemic, isolation and crazy government guidelines limiting their ability to meet and collaborate in the normal way. I must say, I have been very impressed by their joint resilience in what have been such daunting times for many. They seem to have defied those predictions on the news programmes that a serious mental health problem would also arise from the pandemic. Maybe it has helped that they are already a bit bonkers, but I believe that this sizeable project has given them a very constructive focus and kept them occupied.

Once more they have combined their experiences to produce a series of poems that are brutally honest and get right to the core of these complex issues. They make it quite clear that there are no simple solutions in this arena of healthcare. The professionals themselves have to tiptoe around with their clients or patients to find an approach that works best and, even then, it can be fraught with unpredictable outcomes. It seems to be very much an iterative process, trying to find suitable therapy for each person. From that point of view, I do rate their efforts in these works because they illustrate the harsh reality of their conditions and management with a mix of sincerity and sometimes rather dark humour. Somehow, they manage to leave a strong sense of hope for the reader in such difficult and unspoken topics.

They have taken a rather different approach with this final volume in the trilogy by deviating into a treatise trying to explain therapeutic approaches to addiction. At the same time, they attempt to show its use as a very loose template for supporting people with other mental health issues. As someone who is very naïve in these areas, I can see the value in encouraging people to talk about their own issues with others who have had similar experiences. I suspect that, in some cases, this might be more helpful than using professional health services!

I would like to say that it really has been a pleasure witnessing these two idiots working together. They have made me smile a lot of the time, although it is tinged with a great deal of sadness when I realise what they have both been through in the worst of their experiences. Sickness, clinics, hospitalisation, homelessness, abuse and arrests – they have faced the lot over the years and it is heart breaking when I try to put myself in their positions. To see how they have turned their lives around is astounding and very heart warming.

The pair of them have been such good friends to each other, and to me, that it feels like we are part of the same family. Like any pair of blokes, they do take the mick out of me for being so naïve but where would they be without a woman to guide them along? They have promised me that this is the final volume but, then again, they are only blokes!

I, and they, hope that the readers will gain both enlightenment and insight as a result of their efforts.

Mary Fingal 2022

Part I

Curtain Call

Did You Try?

Success often begins with failure
Maybe like a soundtrack on repeat
Sometimes you just have to endure
Lessons learned until you find your feet

Still wobbling for quite a long time
Becoming stable takes determination
No trips and not falling back into the slime
Nose to the grindstone brings you salvation

A new life dawning and a bright sunrise
Bringing great joy and deep satisfaction
Through your commitment no great surprise
Avoiding that tendency toward self-destruction

Attitudes change as you seek what is good
Belief in yourself and what you are doing
Like you've been transfused with new blood
Determination brings that new life flowing

In time you look back and wonder just how
That quicksand bog didn't gobble you up
Dwell not but be thankful you are here now
Keep one eye on the ball and never give up

The how and the why don't matter at all
Revel in the present you were nearly denied
We know not of tomorrow so enjoy the ball
Then no-one can say that you never tried

Dodgy Dave

There once was a junkie called Dave
Who liked nothing more than a rave
But one day he slipped up
While trying to jack-up
Now he looks up from his grave

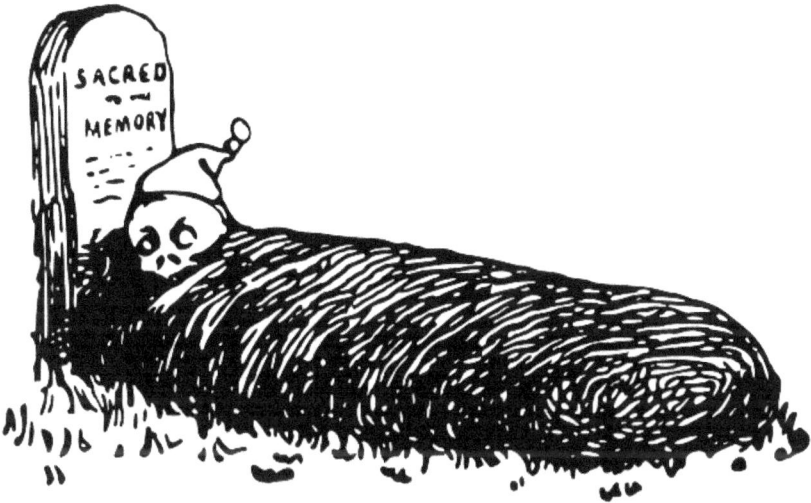

Addicts' Theatre

Addicts make the greatest actors
Fables of desperation and crime
Or "I'm going to get sober this time "
A blatant lie but one we so often believe
Stories of intense hunger begging for food
Though the only food they seek
Is the one they crave in self destruction
They convince us that this is what they need
A tragedy of constant turmoil
Not just for them but for us too
As we watch them writhe in pain
They follow no scripts
Every scene is performed as improv
Moments of comedy are very few
Romance is ugly when you are kissing pills, needles or booze
Talents wasted in live action
The cameras are never off
No directors to say "cut" or edit the final reel
Addicts have a new sequel every day
Though the plot is familiar
They're just great at holding centre stage
One day I know the final credits will no longer show their name

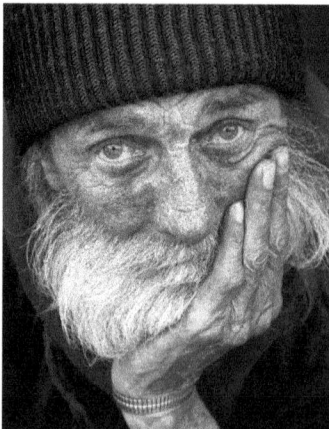

Addicts' Movie

I'm the protagonist in my own personal horror movie
Scene after scene the narcotic band of antagonistic croupiers
Heroin, bourbon, cocaine even suicide were daily battles I faced
In those depths I was merely existing
As I repeatedly climbed those twelve steps
Years of falling down in this intoxicated Jenga
I never believed I'd be alive to see the première
Thought I'd be raven carried before the ending credits
However, I rewrote the script
I've torn up the blueprints and changed the formula
This horror's now a psychological thriller
Even Stephen King will never guess the killer

Comprehensive Corporal

A golden Chevron
With symmetric vines
This insignia
Warranted a rank I fought for
Scattered battles with education
Skirmishes with exam papers
Classroom combat in close quarters
Graded by invisible hands
Merited with nine pieces of eight
A comprehensive corporal
I graduated with glorious promotion
Never valedictorian but no one achieved more
Despite the detention and cliques
I went the distance
The full twelve
I completed high school

Loatland

I have told a thousand tales
Written a million words
About the struggle inside my skull
That chaotic realm
Where every voice is wild like a banshee
This unknown darkness grows
Full of alligator wizards and bloody crocodiles
I'm drowning in speeches
Though it used to be bourbon or rum
A spiralling ladder round the beans talk of insanity
Free falling into pits of fires
Burning scars like piano keys
The frequent trips to Loatland
A carousel of emotions riding the rollercoaster
Shipwrecked among my demons
My daydreams are horror stories
The authorial quill is running dry
I've run out of ink
Just these images inside my crazy mind
A bloody crocodile, an alligator in a wizard's hat
.... I was dancing on the borderline again
It's time to wake up Matt

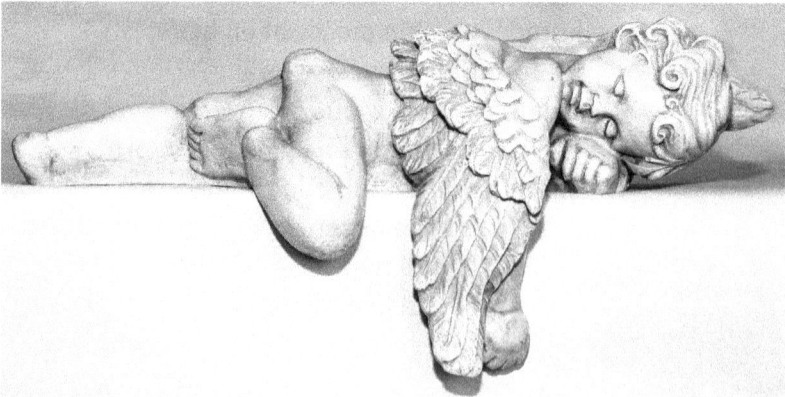

One Way or Another

The acoustic harmonies of wise words
Trickling like a brook against rocks and edges of earth
Every soul we encounter is a teacher
We become their padawan
When you look at your surroundings with true understanding
You will see the beauty
The rawness and nakedness of what's really in front of you
I'm a slut for knowledge
The knowledge to be the best version of myself
Under the microscope of diametric realities of dual power
Karma flows through channels both good and bad
You can change your course and company
If you see the true reflection in front of you
The flaws and imperfections
Alongside your strengths and dreams
I'm a slut paid in opinions and critiques
See more than just what you see
And you'll find a new level of freedom

Recognise your chaos and the need to be changed
Don't let that thirst lead you to over-analysis
Lest the complication leaves you deranged
Keep it simple and you'll avoid the next crisis
Life is a balance between the good and the bad
It needs to swing gently between the two states
Not lurch wildly from one extreme to the other
Simple lessons from both and life's not a bother
Acknowledge your flaws and celebrate successes
You can learn so swiftly to avoid life's excesses
In so doing you can then value your own assets
Don't berate yourself for those mistakes of old
They cannot be changed but you'll learn to unfold
A path to learning the most important lesson of all
To love yourself and avoid that catastrophic fall

Military Mentality

Loaded and locked as I looked down the sights
This unmounted magazine
Vibrates with fire
The emotional bullets ricochet against my skull
Unofficial Marksmen in no man's land
Demon snipers perched in bird nests laid in shadow
My insanity evacuates as a plague upon this earth
Fearlessness doesn't make you bulletproof
Artillery and auxiliary positions mapped out on forgotten blueprints
Camouflaged in the violence and legal murder
Berets bleed in the dust
Will I survive this tour
Aching to see home
Prisoners of cerebral warfare
A holocaust of personal purification
I stand commando to the naked actions I commit
Post-traumatic stress and golden red horizons
Anxiety and paranoia the greatest tools for survival

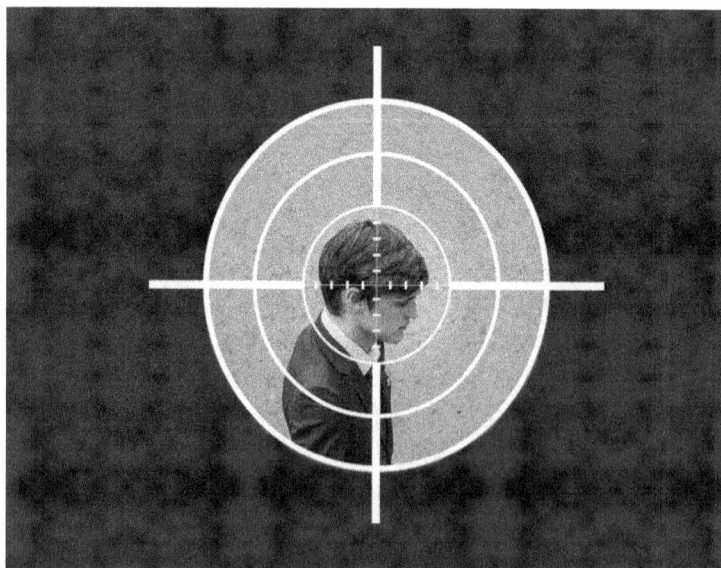

My Confidant

Walk with confidence
Like your Jessica Rabbit
After all this shit
It's time to break the habit
You can be positive
You have a second chance
The band is playing your song
So let's motherfucking dance
It's water over wine and whisky
No more needle games
Wanna see some magic I'm Tricksey
Banksy has nothing on my art
He paints walls and street signs
I overcame addiction bro
Top that bombaclaat
I ain't a harlequin anymore
No longer mute in the wings
Shine that spotlight on me babe
I'm a motherfuckin king

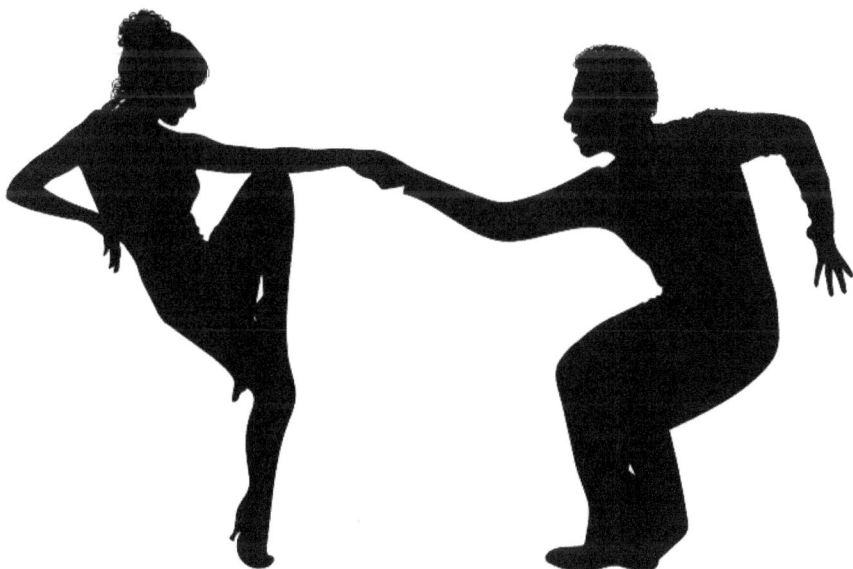

Take Your Time

Curb your enthusiasm my friend
You are nowhere near the end
Just six months under your belt
For years the best you have felt

Early days and you are still just a sprog
You need the wisdom of an old sea-dog
An agility like that of an old mountain goat
These come with time to keep you afloat

Your sense of euphoria we all understand
Temptation to believe that you are a saviour
You are still so fragile as a very new brand
History tells us that haste leads us to failure

We have all seen it happen again and again
The recovery novice trying to lead the charge
Crashing around like an out-of-control barge
Joint relapse inevitable with nothing to gain

So take a back seat, relax and enjoy the ride
Building your resilience as many months go by
A year under your belt, come out of your hide
Cautiously offering support to that new guy

The motto quite simple take one day at a time
Go to bed each night both clean and sober
Please remember your battle is never over
Develop humility and maybe put it in rhyme

Long Walk

It's a long walk home
When you abandoned me at your favourite watering hole
Step after step
Rhythmic drumming on cobblestones
Or submerging in fresh puddles
Once again it was raining
You told me you were "only havin a half"
As you left me on that bench with my panda pop and bag of ready salted
The raindrops hide my tears
I thought this week would be different
Hours I waited for you
The sun is going down
I'm hungry and cold ... but you weren't coming back
Peeking through the smoke stains on the window
All I saw was your potion in your hand
Surrounded by your glass necklace
I covered many miles as I went walkabout
The door to our hovel was locked
So I slept on the steps
I never woke up
They said it was pneumonia
You stayed to the bell
We both heard last call
Now which regret do you have more

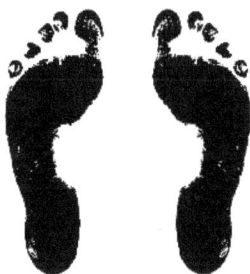

Missed Calls

I used to curse every time you'd call
"Leave me alone "
My daily chants
Quite often I would just watch my phone ring
Practising my cricket bowl
The rectangular ball slams hard against my homely surfaces
Forever turning the volume down
Surfing silent conversations
I plead continuous ignorance
But now I wish the phone would display your name
I'd give anything to see that green button
My keypad of regrets is embedded in my fingerprints
I'm sorry I didn't appreciate the nightly calls
Now it's all too late
Heaven doesn't have a pay phone

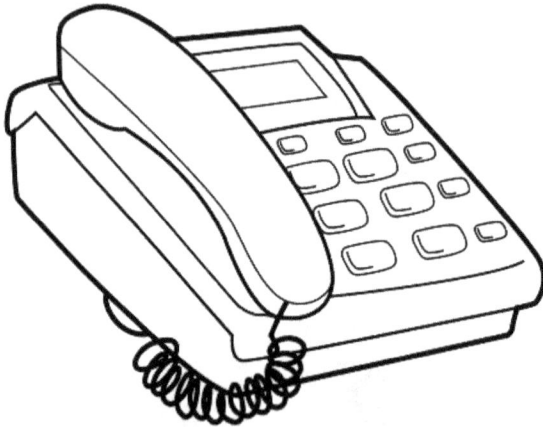

Pocrescophobia

They asked me
Why don't you eat aren't you hungry
The truth is yes I am
I'm also scared
My insecurities binge on every bad feeling or thought
Disgusting FAT gross
I've been called them all
Many times my nachos were seasoned with tears
Magnums taste different when flavoured with guilt
I love food but food hates me
The sweet chocolate cake scent in my apartment
Makes me gain ten kilos just thinking about it
Friends say I'm beautiful
The mirror says different
Triggered by yummy treats
If I have them I'll starve myself for a week
Chronic vomiting after every meal
I will be skinny and pretty
Derailing on all of my curves
Men like my boobs and arse but that's all
Please stop telling me to eat
My stomach is growling so bad it disturbs my sleep
Crying at get togethers or in my car
No one judges me worse than me
I survive on water and salad
Even that is hard
It's an eating disorder
My on-going nightmare
Counting calories in everything
Hiding in hibernation
Please understand food for me is traumatic
I wish I could lose weight
The scales needle is static

Invisibility

I have an invisible illness
There are quite a few
BPD, fibromyalgia, depression and bipolar
They're real but you can't see them
You see the scars on our arms
Or the days we can't leave our beds
Just thinking we are lazy or attention seeking
How wrong you are
It's hell the internal fire of the pains we go through
The screaming voices in our heads
Juggling the mania and manic lows
We push everyone away because we're scared to be alone
Flares of unrelenting agony rip through every piece of flesh
Even the smallest tasks like showering can leave us feeling like death
We wish you could understand
Why we need our spoonies
Or often cancel plans last minute
I'm not trying to annoy you
Please I'm trying to explain
Why invisible illnesses need more people to know
That we are trying our best and please kind
No one ever asked for this
We didn't line up and say give us everything to shut us down
But despite that we fight every day to do normal things live normal
lives
So I hope now you think twice
When that one friend is struggling
You can't see what's going on
They need a hug or three and for you to be supporting

Aficionado

I'm an aficionado of survival
My commodity is mental health
Lost track of the battles with demons
The string of scars on my guitar canvas
The pattern strumming a ballad
My song is a common one
There's millions of us in the band
One voice providing lux in the darkness
A heathen village of cerebral poltergeists
Dressed up in cosplay
Is the man the one who survived the beasts
Or the beast who looks like a man

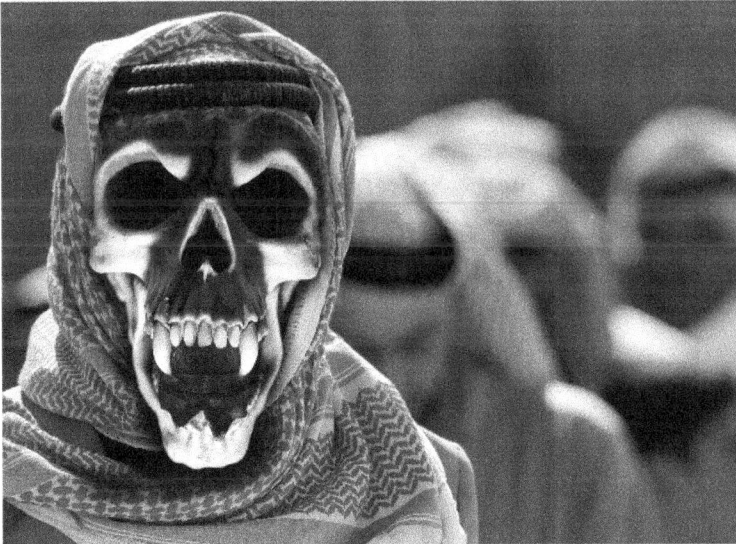

Demonic Attack

The demons took me out today
No not like that ... I'm not writing from the grave
We went to the carnival
Started on a rifle range
Every time I hit a target I pretended it was you
Hook a duck for a prize
Teddy bears and fluffy unicorns just hanging there
Tee'd off in mini golf
Through the windmill .... nope
Evil clowns laughing at me
Try again for that hole in one
Nope the Tiger Woods style isn't working
Fuck it let's go Happy Gilmore .... ping
Hitting the freeway counts right
Oh look a candy stand .. whoops wrong sort of candy
Drunk tank sorry dunk tank the meds make reading hard
Baseball pitch and .... bullseye the hobbit goes swimming
This is fun
Oh bugger I'm missing a voice wait there he goes
Into the room of mirrors
Wow everyone says the reflection is funny but mines perfectly
normal
This is how I always see myself
Wow bumper cars at least I don't need a license to drive these
Ok Matt channel your inner Paul Walker ......
No that was your inner Mario
What's next
Indoor bowling or claw machines
Hmmmmm oh look a pool table let's go swimming
Arghhh attack of killer cues
Haha en garde motherfucker I'm Bruce Lee no I'm Batman
I don't believe it I'm worthy I've found Thor's hammer
So many stalls with so many colours
I'm standing in a painting

The smells of doughnuts and beignets
I wanna go on all the rides
The rollercoaster, the water ride, spinning tea cups
The haunted house no no I'm not ready to go home no
This is a kaleidoscope of craziness
I think I'm gonna like it here

Supernatural Night Fever

All alone on a Saturday night
Just the anticipation and silence
They're coming for me, my children and grandchildren
This watered-down whisky offers little comfort
I've seen this happen before
The bastards took my mother away
Jack-knifed into a realm of supernatural fears
Across the bridge at night
I'll give them a welcome
Worthy of Dean and Sam
I know it's all in my head .... isn't it
If this is just another hallucination ......
Then where did this Winchester come from

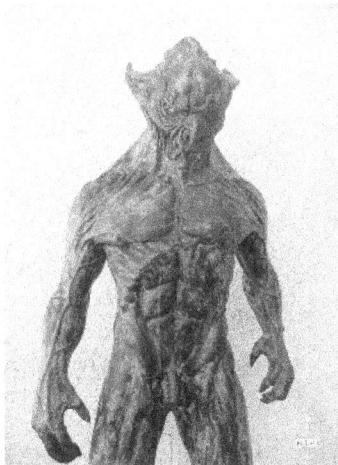

Choices

When drink and drugs
Brought out the worst in us
Decisions made
A thousand mistakes
It all fell apart
Left you alone in the dark
Raise the captain's flag
Or take that final drag
From reality we flee
The demons are chasing me
Hurdling fences
Dropping fifty pences
What I'd give to be free of this
In recovery or contented bliss
I can be
If I believe in me
My choices were wrong
I knew it all along
No more running I'll stand and fight
One day at a time just be sober at night

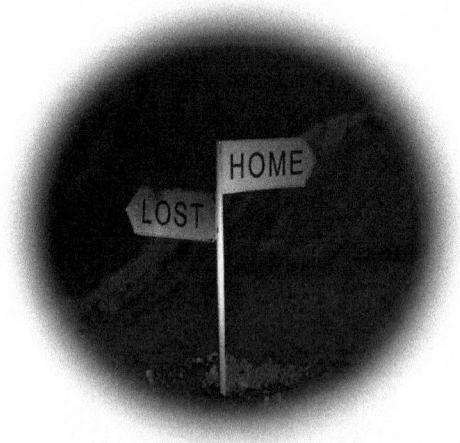

Once Upon a Time

You told me
All dogs go to heaven
I watched as the last unicorn disappeared
Nana always called me her brave little toaster
In this land before time
There was Biker Mice from Mars
We had conversations with talking chocolate stars
At home in the gum trees
With skippy the bush kangaroo
Pete had his dragon
Emerald green and pink
The Chitty Chitty Bang Bang of cars passing by
Imprisoned weekly in Fort Boyard
The swimming classes with Flipper
Jumpin Jacks and art attacks
Often we camped out in the mud
Is it any surprise that I went insane
When this was my childhood

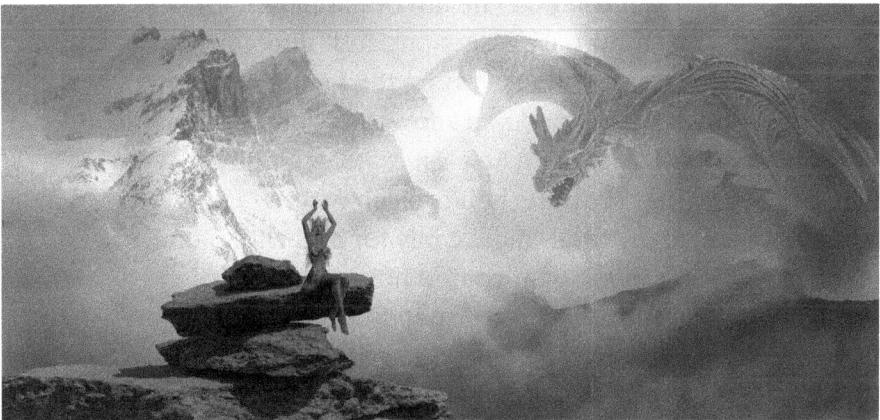

A Plea

Please don't judge a book by its cover
For the addict or mental health patient
A human being wanting to get better
Needing support not sarcastic lament

You may never understand them fully
But please don't just turn into a bully
That simply does nothing for anyone
Creating anger when there need be none

The best thing you can do is encourage
Support from professionals and peers
For the sufferer it requires some courage
Yet the benefits will last many years

Man Made Money

Money, cash, wonga, funds or brass
Whatever you call it .... it's fake
It can't buy health or happiness
Just material possessions and fuckin drugs
I've wasted thousands on the high-end candy
Drink rivers dry and had snowball fights with Charlie
Cash is king no cash is a commodity
That supports habits laced with insanity
How many times did we pay for pills with pennies
Or burn sugar coated fifty-pound notes
Those needs for speeds were strong
Fuck the bank and wallets empty
Drug dealers don't accept pebbles or pleas
Credit isn't an option
So it's back to begging on the streets
Where did it all go wrong

I had it all
Pregnant wife and unborn daughter
Family car, a holiday home
My life used to be in order
Now it's scattered like Lego across infant carpet
Pockets full of lint and empty air
I finally realise just how much wealth I had
When I had people who gave a shit in good times or bad
It was me
I went to the track with the savings
Backed a horse who's still running
The whisky therapy seemed a safe escape
All I did was open a room of mirrors and doors
I don't know the way out
Spent years married to addiction
Now I long for divorce
I've paid the price
My ticket wasn't golden it was artificial
Too long did I play a losing hand
I'm getting my life back
And I'll do it bankrupt and alone
From Bentley's and a four-bedroom house in London
To a gypsy road and a broken-down mud-stained caravan
I'm home

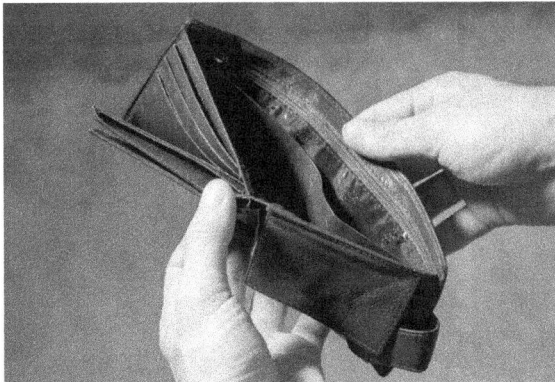

The Fighter

I've always been a fighter
A gypsy kid boxing in car parks
Brawling bare knuckle outside church
I was forever in trouble
Trained hard and honed my skills
Day after day wrestling with thoughts
Who knew my hardest fight would be against myself
From a black belt in Kickboxing to a black belt in depression and anxiety
I'm a broken beat-up wreck
The bad days leave me burning
I cut, I bleed .... damn I can't stop hurting
Bloody faced and battered hands
My hearts turned black I don't feel fuckin human
I'm trapped in my head
This cerebral cage is the pavement arena
No one else to blame
This self-inflicted violence
You are blind to my opponent
I'm not alone
Stuart is laughing at me
My own personal Gollum
I've broke the first rule of Fight Club
Go ahead send me to Tyler Durden
You can't hurt me anymore
I'll survive this storm
I'm not scared of getting knocked down
Coz I'll get right back up
No matter what I'm going hell to leather
"One more round "
Just keep telling myself
"Go one more round "
Let's have it motherfucker
Guess I was born to be a fighter
Always and forever

To the Dogs

I was a seventeen year old pup
Running with the hounds after the hare
Our Harley's made the tarmac shiver
Leather vests and patches on my chest
Empty beer bottles every night
Decked out in black and yellow
Slutty women and an open road, I was corrupted
A non stop two years of partying
We paid our dues, the bar was always stocked
Weekly church around the table
Every time the gavel hit the glasses were its encore
A clubhouse full of debauchery and beer-soaked matrimony
All revved up with my brothers and bitches
Brawling like a Bulldog or acrobatics with Antelopes
There was never a dull moment
I was riding fast and living free
From a foot soldier to the sergeant
Always I'd answer the call to arms
Then It all went to the dogs
Betrayal, fratricide without the killing
Brothers fought and blood was spilled
The bullshit and bollocks was too much
Perhaps it was always like that
I was just blind on beers, bourbon and false brethrenhood
Now I'm alone riding nomadic roads to nowhere
We all said "ride or die" .
Safe to say it's dead now with no resurrection
For two years the DOGS MC left its mark
No longer will we bite and this was 'pups' last bark

Mouldy Junkies

Do you remember, my love
We used to share needles and a cockroach ridden mattress
Starving
For our narcotic groceries
The brown paper bag was our bible
A lifetime of pawn, porn and theft
I wish I could hock my memories away
Every time I look at my 'track' record
I see the human stilton of mouldy veins
A reminder of our darkest moments
...... but now we share banquets of smiles and laughter
Bowls of cereal and Shepherd's Pie
Our new bible is the album of photographs
The new adventures of running along the brook
Camping on beds of ferns and pine cone pillows
The blinding warmth of the morning sun
No longer do we live like rats in shadows
The night still comes
Let it
.... I'm not afraid of the dark

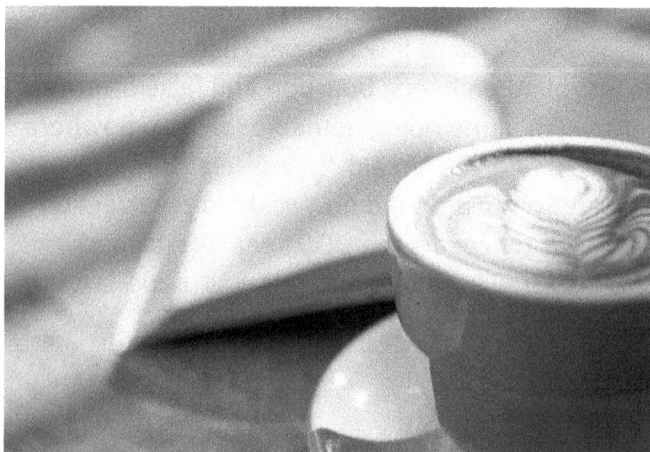

I Woke Up Today III

I woke up today
After years of cerebral conflict
No more pain or anxiety
At peace with my sweet demons
I finally woke up today

Why? III

I woke up yet again
With a real purpose in life
Caring for another so frail
Staying safe in difficult times
Keeping busy and doing good things
To bed each night knowing I've done right
What a joy it is to wake up next day

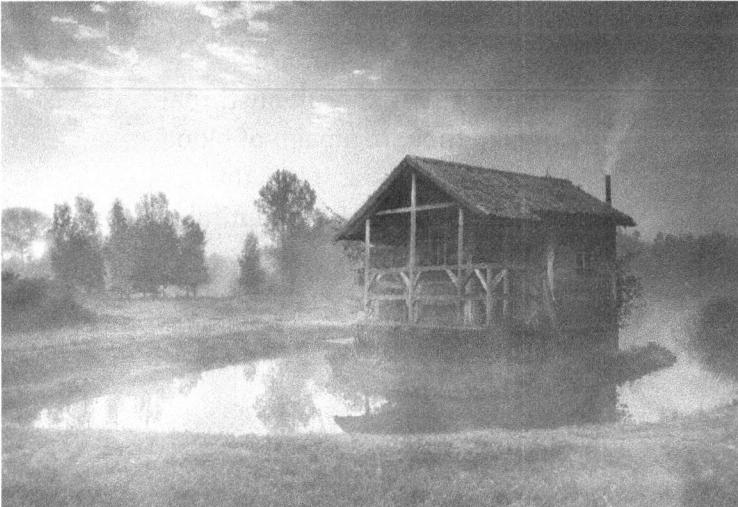

Alone in the Dark

I hid in the darkness
Of this cold hotel room
I can see my breath in front of me
Gentle whispers coming out of the walls
I'm scared
The loneliness leaves me tharn
A shredded bible by my side
Little comfort to be found in those verses
I feel numb to my depression
No sleep
The Devil's marooned me in his playground
A scratching pierces the silence for a moment
I thought I heard screaming
But I'm the only one here
Aren't I
The heavy weights of fear pin me down
No light no warmth
The anxious beating of my heart is the only sound
There's something in the woodwork
My imagination is manifesting a portal to a very real Hell
I'm in a nightmare
I close my eyes as I rub my throat
Opening them to a palm of blood
A silver kiss stings as it hits the floor
The concierge has such a beautiful smile
I'll rest now love
If I need you I have you on speed dial

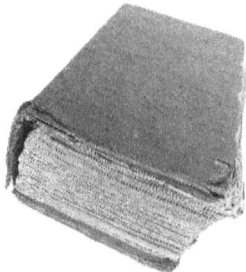

Steve Irwin

In the Queensland sun I dream
My residence a castle in the swamp
Indigenous songs played on eucalyptus strings
I swim with crocodiles in a waltz
On muddy lands or in the outback sands
The red rock heart is beating
Chasing dingo or kangaroos
Cuddling with a koala at Australia Zoo
A shadow in the mirror
In the moon above the ocean
The insanity of a man's passion
Thousands of stars their eyes still burning
My dream time tribute to a legend
Sleep well my friend Steve Irwin

Dedicated to the memory of the late great Steve Irwin whose passion matched our own insanity
RIP Steve Irwin

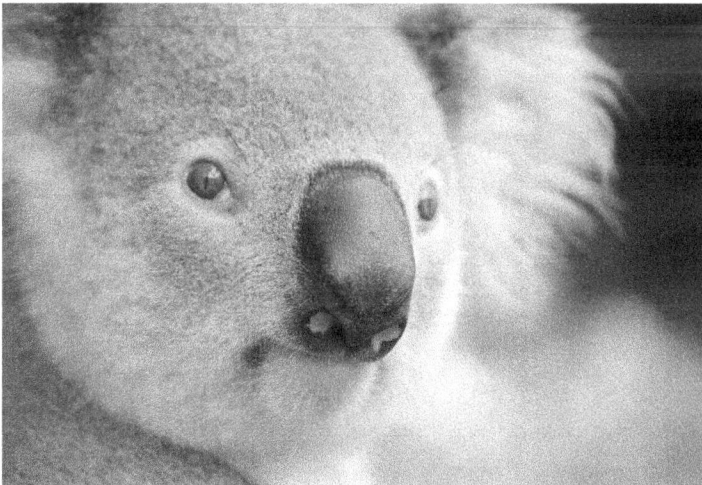

My Musical Episode

The bayou chorus is singing to me
Loup-garou ripping on the harmony
Vampire acoustics with a vibrating voice
Down in the moonlight there's a hidden noise
Coz I wrote this song without the lyrics
It's the melody that you can hear
And I'm blazing baby like a firefly
The stars are dancing in the sky

Alligator wizard he does the tango
My doppelgänger drumming while I'm playin' the banjo
Witches are brewing up some magic potions
A coven of supernatural devotion
Heretics believe they can...can....can
The real monsters are the mortal man
Birds and beasts coming from afar
To get down and boogie in our Mardi Gras

The bayou chorus is singing to me
Loup-garou ripping on the harmony
Vampire acoustics with a vibrating voice
Down in the moonlight there's a hidden noise
Coz I wrote this song without the lyrics
It's the melody that you can hear
And I'm blazing baby like a firefly
The stars are dancing in the sky

Forgive me Father for I have sinned
It's been weeks since my last confession
I've hurt so many people
With my words and ignorance
Living too much in the past because I'm scared to move on
I can't accept others compliments or encouragement
Forever in betrayal of my own mind

Part I - Curtain Call

Only counting my failures
I don't think I'm good enough
The great alligator wizard still weighs heavy on my mind and heart
Drunk daily on the bad juju brewed deep in bayou water
I no longer believe God can save me
Binging on junk food and Daim bars
Pushing the one I love the most away
My scarred arms are seducing me to reintroduce them to the fangs
Internal tears haemorrhage in my soul
I don't want to go on
For these and all the sins of my life I'm sorry

The bayou chorus is singing to me
Loup-garou ripping on the harmony
Vampire acoustics with a vibrating voice
Down in the moonlight there's a hidden noise
Coz I wrote this song without the lyrics
It's the melody that you can hear
And I'm blazing baby like a firefly
The stars are dancing in the sky

I'm lost
The great alligator wizard
You left me behind
In this bayou
My tears fall cold
Like shooting stars in a blood red sky
I'm afraid
Of the necromancy and blackness
Your smiling knives were the light
Purple potions upon the shelves
My master's grimoire is torn and tea stained
The unrivalled skills in cartomancy
Lightning and thunder trapped in your sphere
Fog crawls
Faes, loup-garous, vampires are all in mourning

Poetic Symbiosis III

The lullabies of the fireflies are filled with sorrow
Your heir's heart is broken
Great alligator wizard
The sun will be grey tomorrow
Goodbye Father

The bayou chorus is singing to me
Loup-garou ripping on the harmony
Vampire acoustics with a vibrating voice
Down in the moonlight there's a hidden noise
Coz I wrote this song without the lyrics
It's the melody that you can hear
And I'm blazing baby like a firefly
The stars are dancing in the sky

Here's my coup de grace
I'll never burden you with my words again
No more chapters in the fable
You can close the book
Finally, the alligator wizard will have some company
Goodbye to the bayou, it's nobility and beauty
Fire choruses in the bell towers of every city I know
I lived
Outside of the corruption in that oubliette
No more words to speak
Time for the white dragon to close his eyes and sleep
Let lightning whip the skies
Give me the death of a warrior poet
Burn my body to ash
Then scatter me in the winds
When the clouds turn black ask the loup-garou to sing
Once more I'll be their audience
The harlequin watching in the wings
And so my story ends
Now yours ....

.... your story just begins

The bayou chorus is singing to me
Loup-garou ripping on the harmony
Vampire acoustics with a vibrating voice
Down in the moonlight there's a hidden noise
Coz I wrote this song without the lyrics
It's the melody that you can hear
And I'm blazing baby like a firefly
The stars are dancing in the sky

Life, Camera, Action

From the rowdy lanes of my council estate
To the peaks of the highest mountains
I've seen sights even hidden to the Gods
There's a trail behind me
Not of breadcrumbs or stones
No houses made of chocolate and sugar
A legacy of mistakes and brawls
In the tread of my footprints
I leave fables, stories and lessons
Is reality any different to a fairy tale
Are those fellow children of my past not also lost
The girlfriend whose eyes melt your heart
Is she not a beautiful princess
Or the handsome prince
The man who holds you against his chest
Protecting you from thunderstorms
Do we not face evil Queens and follow white rabbits
Or justify our acts of piracy and theft
Those we love give us clemency and pardons
The looking glass isn't a portal to far off realms
Instead its a portal to see the soul and scars in mortal women and
men
How many of us are bandits and rogues
Witches and wizards with runes and talismans
We are the authors of our own paths
In your hand rests the quill
Every day a blank page to dance, sing and fill with laughter
Be a hero or a villain
Are you brave enough and true of heart
To write another's and perhaps even your own
...........happy ever after ....

Beautiful Black Beast

The cold barrel pressed hard against my temple
There's no one here to stop me
All the loneliness can be over
I just have to pull the trigger
ONE .... TWO ....THREE
.... the fuckin safety catch is on
I can't even do this right.......... but
Maybe there's .... a reason
Perhaps I'm not as alone as I thought
This silent black beast
He could have released a golden stallion
To stampede straight through me
I feel strangely calm ...... its alien
Deep breaths
No longer do I see the graveyard mist
I don't want Shachath's kiss
Its not my time to walk with the reaper

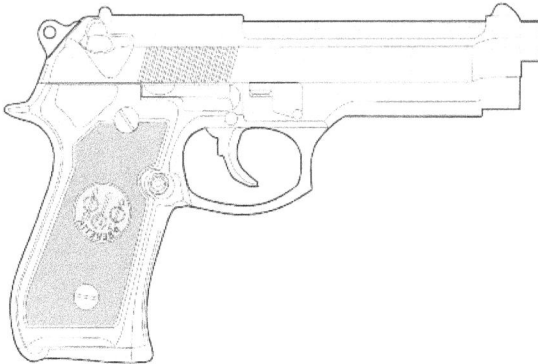

Addicts' Monopoly

The life of an addict
Is a human monopoly
There's buying and selling
Occasionally you'll take a trip to jail
To your personal hotel suite
The in-game debts so high they rival reality
Chests upon chest of paper treasure
Second chances a-plenty
An old dog who can't be taught new tricks
Communities of desperation and disappointment
Always on the move
Never passing go
Simply destined by the roll of the dice

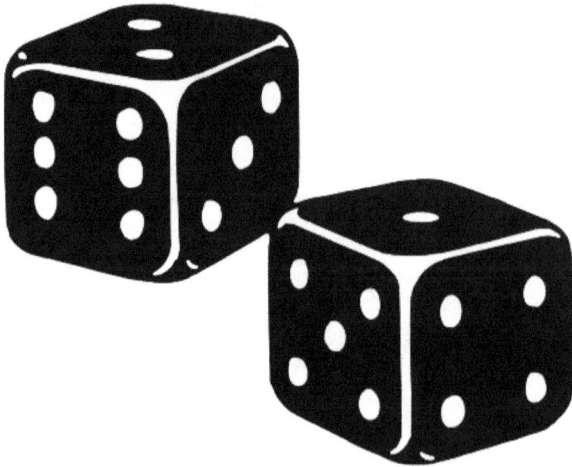

Wakey Wakey

I wake up every morning to an alarm at five
Ever, ever punctual, I'm so glad to be alive
Not like it used to be when I was at my worst
Waking up at any time with a dreadful thirst

Causing chaos all the time I didn't give a damn
Hopeless and helpless my life was just a sham
I knew I really had to change before I hit the meths
Then be another statistic in the register of deaths

Onwards and upwards was what I wanted most
With good support from others, I am not a ghost
My quality of life is now in the first division
Not seen by others as just worthy of derision

Now I wake up with a much more positive view
It has its ups and downs but that is nothing new
No more ducking and diving pretending I am fine
If I'm feeling lousy, I have a damned good whine

Keeping busy is the secret to my own success
Doing good things stops me getting in a mess
No looking back in that stupid romantic way
Glad that time is over as I get on with my day

There is hope out there for anyone who is in a state
Don't wallow in self-pity or misplaced arrogance
Wake up now and ask for help before it gets too late
Then you too can have a life like a new romance

As the Crow Flies

I watched a murder
Silent and methodical
A slow creeping mist across the ground
Macabre and depressed
Strokes of emptiness and cold
Pecking as the black paints wash over a midnight purple canvas
Is it strange that I smiled
The blueness of the beaked knives
A subtle voice lingers
Its dialect unrecognizable
Merely whispering into pockets of wind
Oiseaux effrayés in the wings
A hidden crime in nature's song

Aussie Rules

I'm living my life by Aussie rules
Running sixteen steps at a time
Avoiding ghostly bombs and verbal violence
From the Port side these audio howitzers fly
My mental state is trapped in this oval
Wooden birds .... I see wooden birds in flight
Curving freedom in this Coliseum
Singing kookaburra's and crows
The horizon flips her light switch
From coastal sunshine to desert nights
The orchestra of bats linger in the shadows
A trail of red sandy footprints
Once again I stand in fire
The menagerie of wildness calms me
Secret stories in this schizophrenic tunnel
My compass is broken
Starboard palette of sky oceans

Part I - Curtain Call

I'm awake in my dreams
Like Alice in Wonderland
We both followed white rabbits
Now I'm overboard
Clutching to that jagged rope that rips my skin
I'm croc bait
Those yellow eyes stalk me
I'm the big fish on the end of the hook
There's no way home
Monsoon rains lash against the canvas
I'm being watered down
Diluted like a human cordial
The midnight blue in a fishbowl
I can't hold on anymore
The current pulls me under
As I fall deeper
Toward inevitably this watery grave
I hear the whispers of Harry Belafonte's "Dayo"
Daylight comes and now I'm finding Nemo

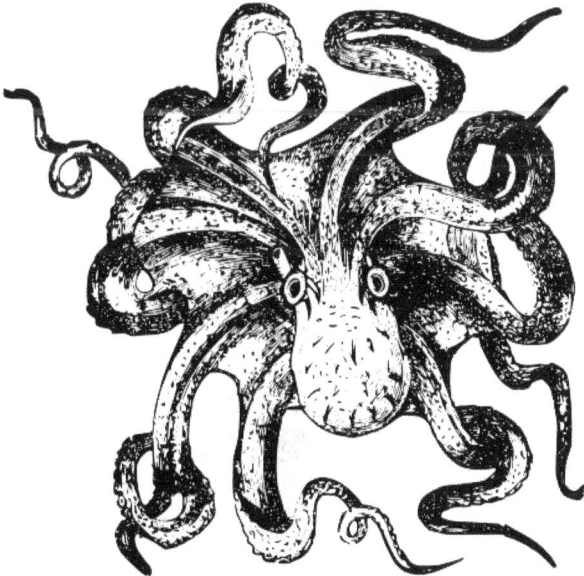

Sin City

Now I cruise my Chevy into Sin City
A fallen star bright in that Nevada Desert
Surrounded by choruses of raining coins
Slot machines of every kind
Mechanical and human
A vibration from multiple toxins
Commodities easily pinballed between tables
Census alive with electricity and endorphins
In pursuit chasing the hare round the track
Pleasantries and subtle gestures among the crowd of peers
Small victories to appease the lust and appetite
Seduced by blind luck and a pretty face
The croupier smiles as she strokes the cards
That roulette of emotions as you realise you've lost
The house always wins
Now the adult entertainment
As you strip away your clothed dignity
Lonely figures wandering nomadic routes
The echo of cheers from the burlesque show
Harsh nakedness of the silent addiction
Tricked into thinking it's just a game
Only to be left in solitaire
With only an empty wallet and a crash course of reality
Sin City the sultry slut .... her light stays on
The Casinos and the Mafia fill their pocket line
Viva Las Vegas baby
The home of legal crime

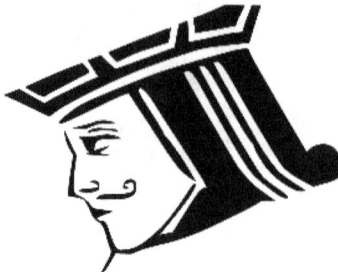

Insane Inheritance?

I've been wrestling with the words
And now I'm under oath
To share my testimony about my mental health
Diagnosed at twenty-seven but the battle had been going on for years
Imaginary friends and conversations with invisible peers
Surrounded by addiction but I wasn't the addict
My mother is bipolar and my father schizophrenic
It was inevitable I would fall into the abyss
Asperger's and Complex Personality Disorder
What the fuck is this
The self-harm and violence
I'm in a nightmare but I'm fuckin wide awake
The voices in my head still plague me shit they get so loud
I want to escape but there's no way out
Some days there is no distraction
Just a pen and paper to record my frustration

Destiny Normal

There is no stain on your character
With mental illness or addiction
Addicts can take actions to recover
In mental illness much greater restriction
Complete elimination maybe impossible
The addict can at least park the problem
Yet it lurks with relapse always possible
Maybe opposite ends of the spectrum
But they have so many issues in common
Mutual support can prevent the inevitable
Allowing normal lives with which to get on

41

Mary's Grog

Mary had a little drink
She also hid a bottle
And everywhere that Mary went
The grog was sure to go

She staggered into work one day
Which was against the rule
It pissed the boss and workers off
To see her act the fool

And so the boss he chucked her out
But still she hung around
Waiting patiently for her snout
To buy another round

Then he grabbed her by the arm
Quickly dragging her away
Saying "Time for the funny farm"
"Rehab is now the only way"

Six months down the line
Now as sober as a judge
She is doing just fine
And resolve will never budge

Inspired by "Mary's Lamb" by Sarah Josepha Hale (1830)

Addict's Lullaby

Rock-a-bye junkie
Sat on the bog
Needle in hand
About to inject
When it goes in
The junkie will fall
And down will fall junkie
Needle and all

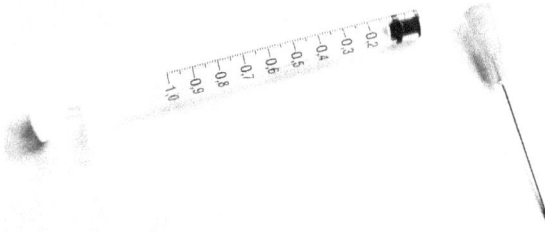

It Was Me

Staring into that stagnant pool
I finally see, I finally accept my reflection
For so long I hated myself, shit I mean I hated the world
Blamed all the bad on everybody else
It was God's fault or I was cursed by some fuckin juju
Thousands of excuses
When in fact ..... I made bad choices
It was me who snuck out at fifteen to go party
I'd drink and fight and fuck like it was going out of fashion
I was out of control
The raging Cajun ....
Getting high on heroin and junk
When I should of been making gumbo and finding a job
Smoking cigarettes like prohibition was coming back
The weed and rocks pulled me in and weighed me down
I didn't do anything to stop myself from drowning
In fact I dived deeper
Mama cried every night her tears filled the bayou
How did I make it this far
Too many of my friends are on the other side
There's fireflies carrying memories to the stars
The bouquet of MoonRoses
Fresh scented flowers on my empty grave
I had the choice
To be buried alive, the walking dead
Broken footprints and blind carnage
Or to see the life beyond the poppy seeds and empty bottles of
Merlot
Black cherry smoke kisses out of the fires in the water
I have to be a man now
Le salaud ne peut pas traverser la frontière

Amber
(Telephonic Salvatore)

That phone call saved my life
You never knew
I was right at the end
Ready to give up
When your name appeared on the screen
It was a sign from above
You spoke to me for hours
Bout everything and nothing
Music, animals, the weather hell even flowers
The distractions you gave me are the reason that I'm here
Crazy that my heroine lives nowhere near
This isn't just a onetime thing
You've saved me so many times all just by giving me a ring
I don't want to die
Now thanks to you I didn't have to say goodbye
You said you would always listen
Even when I was talking rubbish to get my head out it's prison
I can't say thank you enough
What you do for me is a whole new level of love
No matter how bad I was feeling
At the end of our talk you'd have me smiling wall to wall and floor to ceiling
The words to thank you won't come out my mouth
So my deepest thanks to you I'm writing it down
Please if anybody is ever so broken
That they're running to the end
Pick the phone up reach out to your family or friends
They really do love you and they really do care
You don't have to do this alone anymore mon cher
One more time you saved me thank you
My friend, my heroine and my Amberooo

Dedicated to Amber Elizabeth Crowe, a valued friend

The Long Run

My journey's been a thirty-year marathon
I've had nightmares and sweet dreams like Marilyn Manson
Mental health left me black and blue
But it made me a champion
After all the abuse and abandonment I'm the last man standing

Who's Boss?

You are not the master of your own destiny
There are many factors beyond your control
Your choices affect its direction and harmony
Although there can be no guaranteed goal

Adaptability in your life path is essential
With both successes and errors along the way
Errors are human and also educational
Not simply failures and a reason to stray

Life may not always go the way you want
It might be a sign of something you need
Not self-destruction but look to the front
No dwelling in regret, on the present you feed

Hope is a four-letter word not to forget
Not like the one we so often prefer
Positivity not arrogance is the secret
Always remember that you're the gaffer

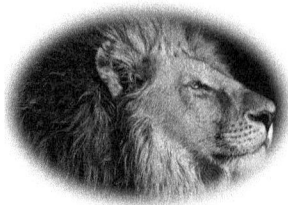

Wedded Abyss

It didn't work
Why didn't it fuckin work
Stop laughing at me
You married me
With woollen handcuffs and two rings
One for the branch above ten feet high
The other for my throat
We said till one of us dies
You left me hanging
Like I was merely a human chain
Swaying across your chest like a pendant
The fuckin branch broke
I failed again
Now all you do is laugh
I hate you I hate you I hate you
Great now it's raining
What's that ..... a shadow in the mist
An amber silhouette in this waterfall
There's a softness on the wind
I'm being watched
I can hear you
Have you always been here
Was I just deaf to your voice
There's a message on the Anna Banana coloured gate
I can hear your voice
You said
"You're gonna be alright mate "

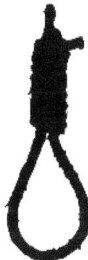

Recovery Ride

Recovery can be like riding a rollercoaster
Maybe many more than one peak and trough
With extremes of fear and joy, getting faster
Wondering whether you will ever get off

The final stretch levels, slowing right down
A return to normality and a stable life
A great sigh of relief lifting that frown
At peace with no need to repeat that strife

But be on your guard all of the time
That fairground is never very far away
Sounding like fun but it's really a crime
Its distorted music tempting you to stray

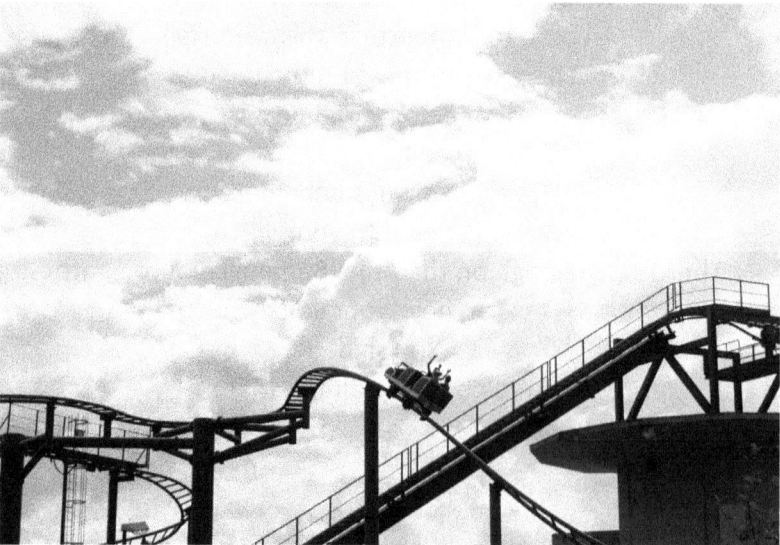

You Too?

Success in recovery is like changing your trade
From plumber unable to switch off a distillery tap
To electrician rewiring cerebral circuits mis-made
A soupçon of psychology and you deal with the crap

Patience and Perseverance the names of the game
No instant fix, each day seems very much the same
The change happens so gently you seem unaware
Maybe some setbacks but in time you will get there

The freedom and joy that you lost will slowly return
All aspects of your life will take on new meaning
Waking with positivity each and every morning
Months and years go by and still lots to learn

Your mood and attitudes become more positive
A real purpose in life develops and gives you a lift
Just keep yourself busy and you won't go adrift
Stay on the right side, you have so much to give

The new life you entered rewards all of your work
Reaching a new normal that makes you feel great
Memories of a past life when you were simply a berk
Treat them with respect, shut away they're just bait

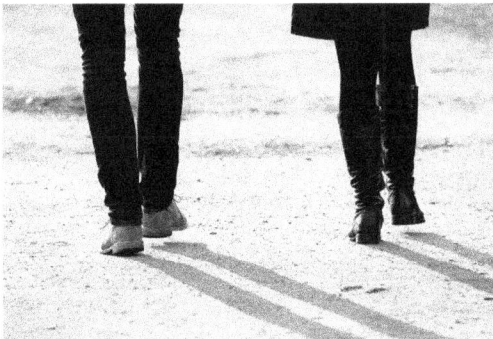

Quaestio Enim

"To be an addict or mental health patient?"
That is the question we would ask you
"Which is worse and which can you cure?"
The question you might ask in return

Your answer to ours would be "neither"
The same as our response to yours
Once developed both are with you forever
From birth, or later, leaving you on all fours

Treatment of either is a minefield
The patient might take drugs forever
For the addict the answer is never
Simply their best and only shield

The patient is permanently haunted
Episodes in a manner making no sense
Medication alone is so limited
It's more of an art than a science

With practice the addict succeeds
Haunted only by temptation or craving
Learning to avoid them serving their needs
Awareness preserves their very being

Yet situations arise where both co-exist
Mental illness leading to addiction
Or vice versa for those who persist
For either there is no perfect solution

Each day we just do the best that we can
All we ask is you neither judge nor condemn
Please remember they are all only human
You too could easily become one of them

A Message

Alcoholics and addicts you're lucky
Recovery grants you your freedom
No more controlled by your Chucky
So welcome to the sobriety kingdom

Not so for the mental health patient
Controlled using substances not for you
Ever haunted, it leads to ongoing lament
Their demons at random out of the blue

With them forever, no turning it around
Yet you can still all support each other
Since you do share some common ground
In that they are like your sister or brother

Always judged by the rest of society
That simply reflects its own naivety
None of these conditions has any respect
Anyone can easily become a social reject

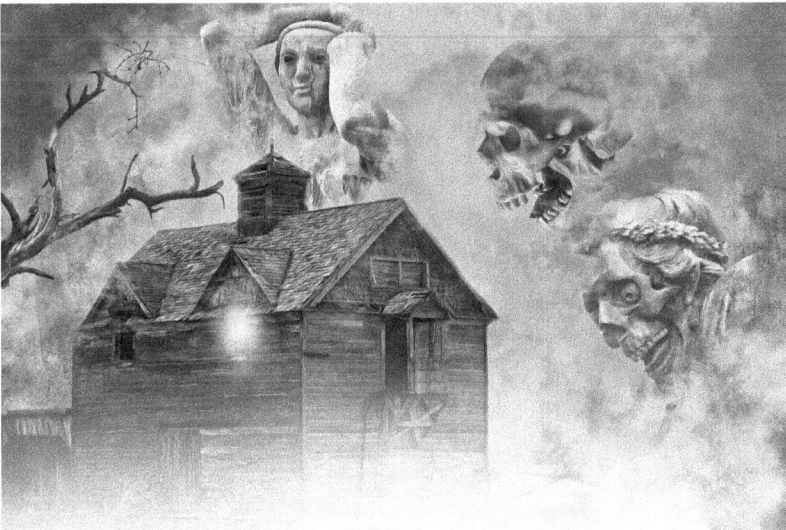

Mutual Aid

Alcoholics and addicts are weak willed
My endogenous depression is an affliction
The drugs I use daily my solution
With their habit they will be killed

Yet I find that I must take my medication
Does that mean I have an addiction?
Does it also make me weak willed?
They do stop me from suicide being killed

It seems that we are just polar opposites
Mirror images of each other somehow?
Maybe a bit like the bull and the cow?
Similar conditions yet different appetites?

So many questions we could ask
We really need to talk to each other
Perhaps not an impossible task
Neither should act as the mother

Different psychiatric conditions embraced
What a wealth of experiences explored
In mutual support and understanding
At last we might feel we are winning

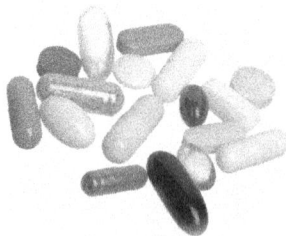

Recovery Theatre?

You wonder why the penny doesn't drop
That switch in your brain won't turn to stop
A serial relapser, a hopeless dead loss
You might just as well not give a toss

WRONG

You are a serial trier, not destined to fail
Each relapse a lesson not happenstance
The dry bits rehearsals for telling the tale
For that final word-perfect performance

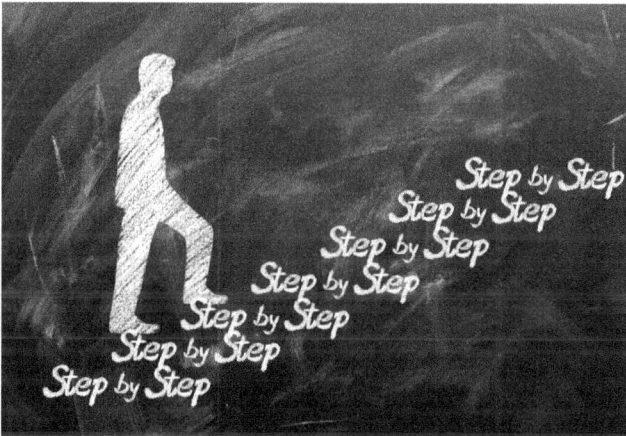

The Journey

There is hope on the horizon
Coming closer if you can just try
Mind-focus requirement number one
No more dwelling in that self-pity

It's time to come to your senses
Learn from your own experiences
Listen to others who've been there
With knowledge of what to beware

Seek professional help if you need to
It can give you a bloody good start
It comes to an end then you depart
No, it's not like a dose of the flu

Ongoing support is so necessary
To keep you on the right track
Sharing experiences good and hairy
Helps avoid the unexpected attack

Being among others like-minded
Not by your success being blinded
Yes, it is truly a lifelong condition
Kept at bay by your own expedition

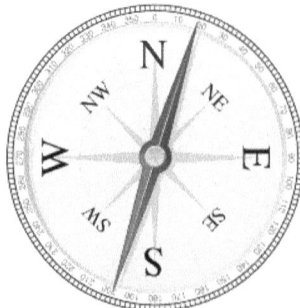

Kill the Switch

Friday night in with the voices
Sat on the couch with my holy water
They keep getting louder and louder
Telling me I'm a burden
Trying so hard to drown them out
I don't want to go outside
The fuckin off switch is broken
Parasites are feeding on my soul
Why won't they stop or sleep
This gnawing is making me bleed
The rulebook hasn't been written
It's Vale Tudo anything goes
A cerebral street-fight in the cranium arena
Outnumbered and armed only with my primitive fists and GTT
I'll go down swinging invisible punches
I can't get buried in this cavity of depression
There's more to me than the darkness
I can turn the lights back on

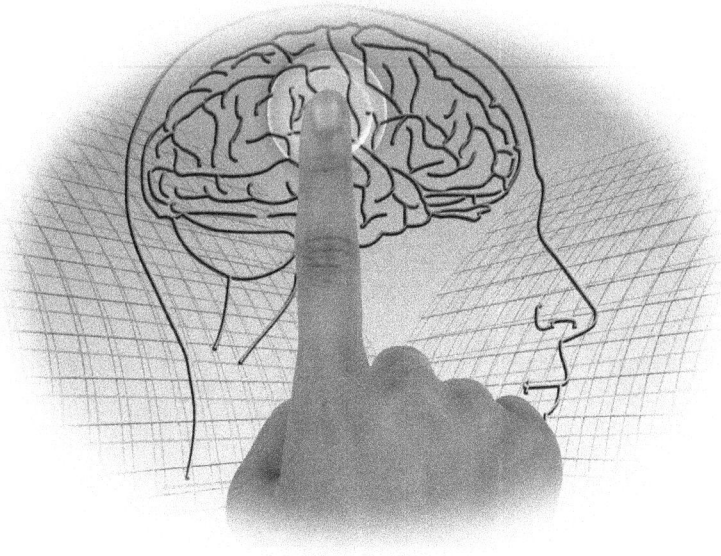

Positive Attitude?

Life in lockdown can be so tough
Television tells us so often enough
"Your mental health will collapse"
"Addicts you might well relapse"
"Mental health patients a total disaster"
Such crap will just make it much faster

It doesn't have to happen even in solitude
So, gird your loins with positive attitude
Keep your mind active with plenty to do
Days all the same but you're not in a stew
Take up a new hobby maybe something indoors
It's got to be better than just cleaning the floors

Any distractions worth their weight in gold
Too much telly news stops you being bold
Stick with programmes that make you smile
Failing all else take a walk or run for a mile
Anything that stops you developing a frown
Just don't let those bastards grind you down

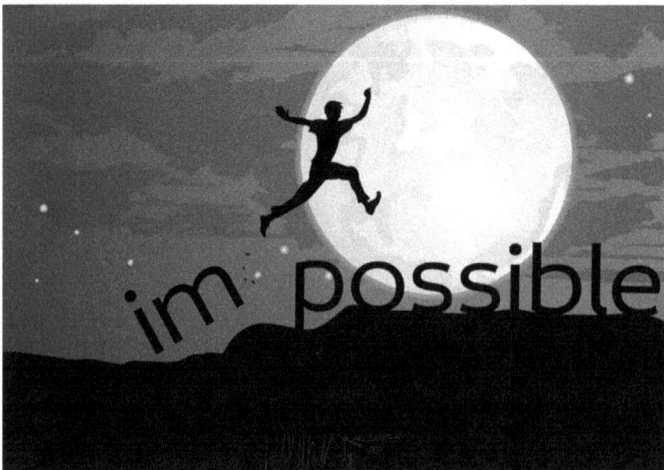

2003

I'll never forget that Sunday afternoon
Way back in 2003
Glued to the square in a fourth story flat
Three flankers but four crazy fans
Sausage sandwiches and empty beer cans
We were on the edge of our seats
It would all be gone in 26 seconds
Lions and a lioness were set to roar
All shivering with anticipation
Waiting to go over the bar
That was the fuckin drop ...... goal
A camaraderie revelling in drunken glory
That Webb Ellis was delicious
Swing low on that sweet chariot
Now it's time to "tip yo waitress"

Public Transport?

Walking by the bus shelter on a sunny afternoon
Drunks inside gobbing off and waving their arms
Loud mouthed behaviour like wolves at the moon
Thinking they were simply showing their charms
Not at all clever, put quite simply each a buffoon
A brief flash of judgement and I look back at myself
Recognising my history is just parked on the shelf
That momentary superiority needs a slap in the face
It was such a tough journey to re-join the human race
No longer behaving just like an uncontrolled gibbon
So easy to slip back, to my recovery I must hang on
Hoping that they can experience that mental shift
That gives them sobriety as their most precious gift

My Father

My father taught me how to survive
From growing crops and firing shots
He loved me though he didn't say it
Riding bikes over green baize hills
Fishing on the river bank
We shared silent bonds
Hidden smiles when we made honeycomb
Da told me that he's bulletproof
Uncle Dunc said it too
Maybe that's why me and my cousin grew up fearless too
Mum was different
She was quiet like a rose
Always in the background
The co-pilot when we travelled the roads
Rock and roll or reggae
The ultimate playlist
Now dads dancing on the other side
He's waiting by the Carmelite stone
I miss him and feel alone
Da had just one love
No longer would he lay his hat at home
I wish I was like him
That I had his strength
He was a Freeman
A man for his family in the hardest times
From the Loat's battle of Hastings
My fearless father taught me to survive
My beautiful mother teaches me to live my life

Bubbles

I'm forever blowing bubbles
Pretty bubbles of fuckin anxiety
The voices in my head
They're wishing I was dead
So I just write crazy poetry instead
Ramblings of a scared schizophrenic
Everything is just purely psychogenic
Now I'm forever blowing bubbles
Pretty bubbles of fuckin' anxiety

Addict's Four Steps

The problem and solution within you
Four simple things you need to do:
Stop pretending to be a renegade
Drop the fucking fanfaronade
Develop some humility
Show the world humanity

Your so-called trips of nostalgia
Simply a bad dose of rectalgia
That past quite simply disaster
Time to become your own master
Live life to the full and turn it around
Not like Morlocks living underground

Frith's Principle

"What if' and "If only" phrases we all use
Trying to understand what has gone wrong
Questions that merely serve to confuse
No answer to why we feel we don't belong

Lord Frith said "What is is what must be"
In answer to Hazel in Watership Down
Not much help when we want to be free
Simply leaving us with one hell of a frown

While he was talking about desperate rabbits
We are desperate to change our bad habits
Simply our present is a product of our past
So, change in the now in a way that will last

We build a new future one day at a time
One foot in front of the other never in haste
Creating that change as slowly we climb
From pits of despair, time we can't waste

Carving a new future, we have to be patient
Trying to rush it will just end in lament
Building that home one brick at a time
With solid foundations and never in mime

Solid commitment is all you require
Changes not obvious until you look back
To reflect on that life that was so bloody dire
Your happy new life is better than crack

Autistic Creole

You tell me
Pull yourself together
When my days are difficult and dark
I thought perhaps you cared
Now I know it was just a charade
A script you read when I'm a burden
Cups of tea and medication
I've heard them all
All the things to make me better
If only it was that simple
Often my mind speaks in Autistic Creole
A language you'll never understand
Millions of dialects and accents
Can't you hear them
I can
I hear them when I'm sleeping and when I'm wide awake
Fluent in the madness and Cajun rage
I wish you could be me
If only for an hour to see the world through my eyes
Pull yourself together might not be your response
You might see things a little different
Not be so quick to judge
Vous avez une belle journée
Ma chérie
I'll be sleeping in the shadow of my lonely bayou

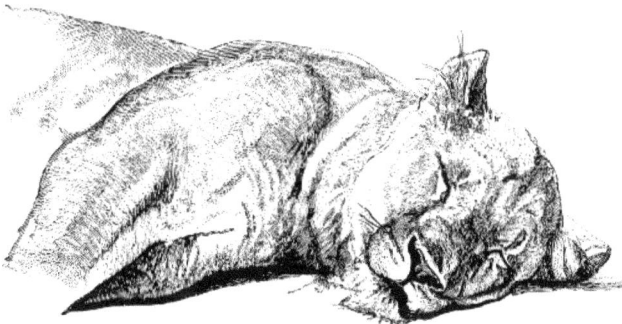

Game of Life

I'm here
North of twenty-eight thousand hours of gameplay
This is real life
The music I listen to daily is my soundtrack
I'm not reading a script I'm living it
Voices in my head get so loud
The reality of hustling these cerebral poltergeists is a struggle
They're playing grand theft auto with my sanity
Trapped in this pressure cooker
At times life has fucked me like I'm a hooker
No protection
Raw and unforgiving
Forever I look for a hiding place
Shelter from the centre stage
A shadow off camera
Or under a quilt of mist in the lonely cemetery
Mental illnesses don't have rules
There's no checkpoint to start over from
Surviving the invisible roads is wild like Donkey Kong
Hurdles barrelling at me from all quarters
Life doesn't have a pause button
There's no such thing as a stalemate
All that's left
Is
Game Over

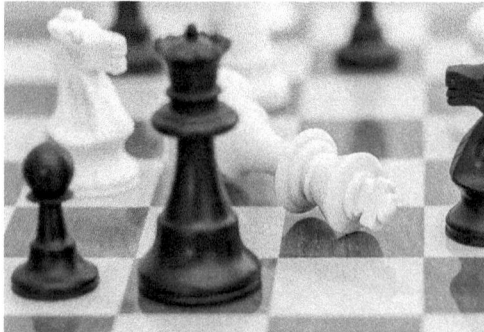

Jack-knifed Johnny

My thoughts are Jack-knifed
Do I carry on the travelling the mental motorway
Or do I crash and burn
There's already been so many twists and turns
Bridges broken and buckled
I've stopped counting the humps and lumps
The bastard cavities have me thrown
Like a feral hamster in her wheel
Cross roads and siren lights
Gridlocked by the cerebral loneliness
As I'm speeding through the canvases
Rural fields and concrete jungles
I used to be safe at the coastal shield
The music has finished
Now my ears are raped by the static audio
Traffic lights dot and dash like Morse code
I'm the only one who seems to notice
Waiting, waiting at this junction in invisible tears
I'm deaf to the bells
Should I stay mute and possum
Here comes the train
Rugged and free
I feel the vibrations through the tracks
The anticipation of inevitable impact
One more glance at the photos on my phone
Any second now
T-boned at the devil's speed
.... the calm blackness fades to grey skies
Guess I'll rejoin the roundabout
My indicators must be broken
I'm back in the wacky races
Once more on El Diablo's highway

Hang Ten

In this rat race we call life
Forever are we chasing
Shadows and dreams
Be us peasants or kings
A chain link of marathons
The constant hustle and bustle
Pixelated faces blurring city streets and tv screens
The world glued in fast forward
Often we forget
The hare set the pace but...
It was the tortoise who finished the race
The beauty painted from nature's pallet
Why don't we stop and take in a view
A pit stop at a waterfall or at a mountain's foot
Before the stopwatch of life starts counting again
Sometimes we gotta go Hawaiian baby
Sometimes you just gotta hang ten

Heaven Sent Hell Bound

I can't do this anymore
Give me the mercy of my final communion
Let the bread be my bullet to the brain
Begging to finally experience the freedom
From my tortured mind
Blood stains as red as the wine I so often slept with
Dreaming in a crimson waltzer
Simply spinning against the pain and abandonment
Here's my act of eternal contrition
Authored a personal sacrament of farewell
Father, Son ....
Now let me become a ghost

Snakes and Ladders

Years following my broken compass
Among the shards of glass spiders crawl
Silence
The very ground of nature has lost its voice
Feral fog swims around my ankles
The piranhas gnawing at the fear in my bones
Each step as tentative as the one before it
The lunar map hidden behind clouds of grey beard
I'm walking deeper on invisible roads
No longer can I see the honeycomb of the labyrinth
My very breath weaved into emptiness
Fireflies trapped in arachnids webs my dimming light
These fears are weighing heavy on my mind
No turns, no exit
Just a growing hunger
Thousands of silhouettes just hanging there
I'm being watched
My stalker is like the chameleon
Camouflaged in capes of blackness
The predator is now the prey
A lonely little boy walking in a man's shoes
That's all I am now
The hairs on my back rise like peacock feathers with every step
Is this the end
Inside the belly of this ethereal beast
I'm at the mercy of this vol de mort
I faintly hear the whispers from my grave
There's a way out from this oubliette of depression and death
It's a game of serpents et échelles
Without the snakes and ladders

The Death Roll

The black crocodile of depression
He has my scent
Submerged in my watery grave
Stalking me in silence
The apex ambush is inevitable
Once more I'll be in the jaws of all I fear
With every bad thought choice .....
I'm being death rolled
There's no escape from this reptilian cyclone
This modern-day dinosaur feeds my tears to his young
My very soul punctured by knife like teeth
Over and over again
The sunlight only adds to my misery

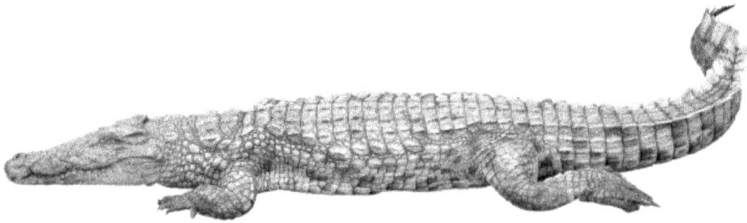

Highway to Hell?

Doing drink and drugs, living easy, living free
Just like in the hit in seventy-nine by AC/DC
You reckon you're taking it all in your stride
But, yes, it's a season ticket on a one-way ride

Things you do have neither reason nor rhyme
Yes, you are simply living on borrowed time
Nothing you'd rather do than enjoy the fun
Like pointing at your head with a loaded gun

No-one is going to stop you or slow you down
Nobody on earth is going to mess you around
Maybe you are just paying your dues to Satan
In spite of that healthy looking but fake suntan

No, it's not an open road but the highway to hell
It will come to an end when Satan tolls that bell
You need to ask yourself one simple question
Die soon or live and try to avoid that destination

That can only be answered by you and you alone
Yes, the choice is yours but make it with care
If life is your choice be like a dog with a bone
Like Special Forces, you can only win if you dare

Inspired by AC/DC and in tribute to Bon Scott, lead singer, who died following a heavy drinking episode

Lithium

Do you hear that farmyard playlist
A podcast of audio telekinesis
Raven's caw and cockcrow songs
Carpet mist crawling like graying arachnids
Lumberjack drums baby I'm lost
In this forest of lumberjack drums

And I'm drowning in lithium
This electric water is pulling me down
Batteries overdosed
Now I'm like a rhino
I'm char char charge charging around
The moon is kissing the sun
Oh baby can't you see me
I'm drowning in lithium

Bipolar twins camped in a tunnel in Paris
Are we dreaming in daylight or just awake all night
My outfit doesn't match and I really don't care
Let's have a cup of coffee love
My ante-meridiem breakfast
Is just like skittles in a bowl

And I'm drowning in lithium
This electric water is pulling me down
Batteries overdosed
Now I'm like a rhino
I'm char char charge charging around
The moon is kissing the sun
Oh baby can't you see me
I'm drowning in lithium

Part I - Curtain Call

Afternoons sat in tears and blackness
Skin on fire with itching burns
Side effects of living in Hulkamania
The ocean of emotions is resting just like a loaded gun
My genie in a bottle whispers my prescription
A lonely existence and a cocktail of misery and bourbon

And I'm drowning in lithium
This electric water is pulling me down
Batteries overdosed
Now I'm like a rhino
I'm char char charge charging around
The moon is kissing the sun
Oh baby can't you see me
I'm drowning in lithium

And I'm drowning in lithium
This electric water is pulling me down
Batteries overdosed
Now I'm like a rhino
I'm char char charge charging around
The moon is kissing the sun
Oh baby can't you see me
I'm drowning in lithium

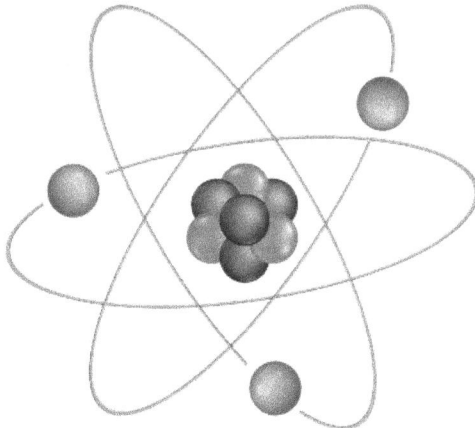

Whose Way?

Like Sinatra I did it my way
I travelled each and every highway
Just because I'd lost the plot
Because of grog I lost the lot
I did it my way

Regrets I have a helluva lot
So many that I have to let go
Or else I would simply rot
So hard to say no
I did it my way

There were times I drank too much
That was like a kick in the crutch
I'd drink it down and throw it up
That was because
I did it my way

No longer loved can't laugh or cry
I've had my fill my share of losing
Time to get a grip no need to die
It's not good
To do it my way

I'm not a man I've lost myself
Time to get off the runaway train
Must ask for help retrain my brain
I have to learn
To do it their way

Pharmaceutical Zombie

I wander
These broken streets
Shards of shattered lights floating in pools of diesel
The aroma of sleepiness
Unbalanced
My medicine is a pharmaceutical zombie bite
I'm alive though I feel dead
Or am I dead but yet still alive
Days when leaving the couch is impossible
I slept through the apocalypse
Thunderstorms of toxicity couldn't wake me
My serotonin levels erratically dance
I'm walking blind even though my eyes are open
I wander
Aimlessly into that open field
That grass stairwell
She spirals onto natures roof
The view is truly beautiful
.... but
Why then am I falling

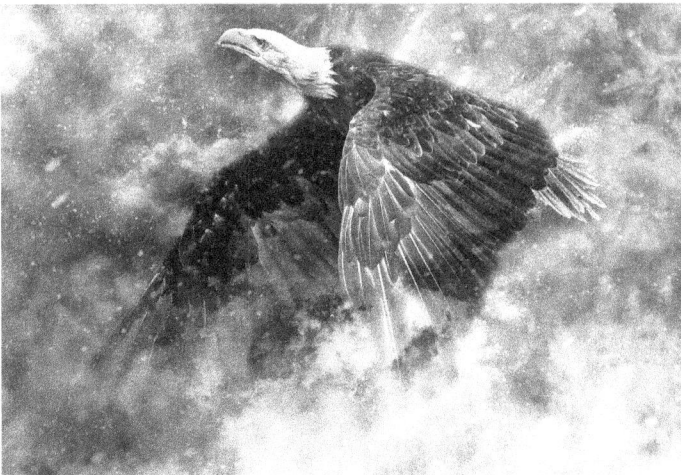

Deal or No Deal

Did I make a deal with the devil
To live freely amongst the webs fractured truths
Unchallenged as I embark on dirty deeds
My invisible vest ...
Merely a sponge for ricocheted bullets against my tarnished soul
The purple bayou hidden deep in Louisiana
She's my personal confessional booth
The alligators and pythons the acolytes of red eyed God
Every word and deed of my memoir is stored there
Every crime and every sentence
The catalogue of détente from family,friends and strangers
The silence now leaves me suicidal
The aching creaks of barks worn down by storms and floods
Fragments .... shards ....
I look above to see a lone astro
She just sits there waiting and watching
The eye witness and accomplice
I spend my days handcuffed in fear and regret
Though my nights are empty smiles as I reread the pages of my
mortal manuscript
Too often I find validation in my outlaw activity
My watery reflection shows a child laughing
In the arms of a man I recognise
Though I left that path long ago
.... now as I bathe in the pardon of hellfire
I etch my story on these rocky walls
The thug who became a writer
Using poetry and song
To tell my gospel of that scared little boy
Whose da taught him to survive
And his mother taught him how to live
Despite all the success and rewards bestowed
I know I don't deserve it

Meeting of Minds

As we sit in this conference room
My consiglieri with their wisdom and counsel
Exploring the avenues of silent debates
I have more questions than answers
The hidden democracy in the mind of schizophrenic men
Lost in crowded rooms
Blind actions lead to unknown destinations
El Padrino of cerebral warfare
The strangest thing
Is my enemies are the same ones
I'm talking too now
Like a family sat in a portrait
The one who isn't smiling
That's the one who's real

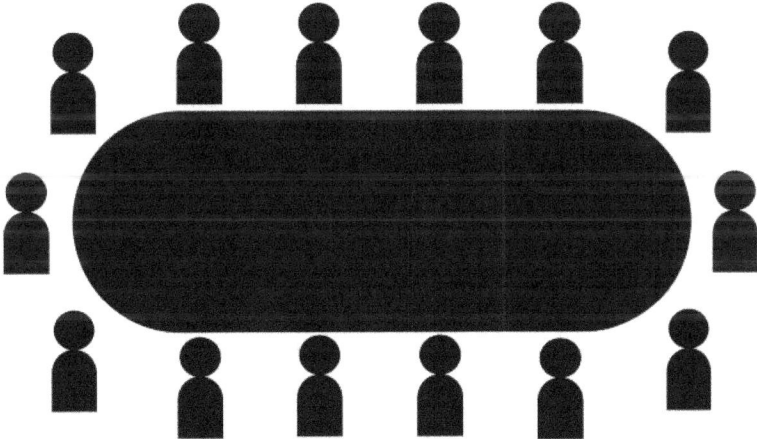

Symbiotic Dichotomy?

Our minds may work in a symbiotic way
Yet there is a dichotomy many may say
One dwelling on things that are negative
The other able to see a life more positive

Expressed in styles that seem so extreme
Vivid and colourful images that need digesting
Compared with a style simple not like a dream
Merging the two at times seems frustrating

The difference may arise from their condition
In mental illness the cause maybe well hidden
In addiction the immediate cause so obvious
Differences in support border on the devious

The addict must abstain from mind altering drugs
The patient no choice but to take those prescribed
A means of control with a concoction contrived
Compared to abstaining and simply not being mugs?

Both groups do require some additional support
Through counselling or groups that write no report
The patient not cured in the true sense of the word
Yet they really can help all of us feel free as a bird

Patients' brain networks not affected by choice
The psychoactive drugs change their internal voice
Just dampened by treatment their world doesn't change
A brain wired differently expressing themselves strange

In addiction abstaining removes an external cause
There remains internal danger that can lead to relapse
Preventable with moral support not drugs of course
Without those mistakes, life so much better perhaps

Allowing the brain to work in a near normal way
We see the world differently like before we fell foul
Unlike the patient whose demons don't go away
We all think and write differently as wise as an owl

In final conclusion we can learn from each other
Working together helps both to move forward
Strengthening resolve without too much bother
Writing wise crap stops each one being a coward

In Memoriam

Dear friend we will all miss you so much
A great ally and an example to one and all
Your support far better than any crutch
Yes, you helped each one of us walk tall

Mixed humour and bittersweet experience
Combined in a manner so gentle yet true
Helping many of themselves to make sense
Making a team out of a motley old crew

No pretence at being an angel or a messiah
Both feet on the ground not head in the clouds
You taught every one of us how to reach higher
How to use humour and not just be clowns

Never to be forgotten by those left behind
Your legacy lives on influencing so many
Recalling you fondly as so good and kind
Carole rest in peace it won't cost a penny

In memory of Carole D, who sadly passed away March 2021

Poetic Symbiosis III

Part II

Therapeutic Symbiosis

A Rational Approach to Therapeutic Support (RATS)?

Poetic Symbiosis III

Foreword

Let's face it, in active addiction everyone has been a rat, causing mayhem for themselves and everyone around them. Please excuse the play on words and the acronym in the title, but they sit well in showing those "opposites" that we encounter throughout life and inexplicably co-exist. What on earth is rational about rats and how can we be rational about irrational behaviour? Acronyms also impress so-called experts in any field.

There are probably as many different pathways in recovery as there are people, ranging from doing it completely alone through to pleading with your god for help. They all have one thing in common in that we seek to change ourselves and our relationship with whatever addictive behaviour we exhibit. "By any means necessary" is a useful motto - if it works for you, do it! Your approach may have a single foundation, but so often we pick and mix the parts that suit us from different theoretical and practical approaches. We are our own experts on ourselves, but sometimes we have to be wary about that lest it leads us on the wrong path – self-will run riot!

This kind of compulsive and often self-destructive behaviour is very complex in its origin at biological, psychological and sociological levels. There is no single or one-size-fits-all model for either its origins or management and the whole topic is filled with equally complex theory and vocabulary. Whilst useful in gaining some understanding, the terminology and theory can be very daunting to the sufferer which, in itself, can have an adverse effect on their engagement in recovery. "It is too complicated for me, so why bother?"

Even a well-educated individual can become a hapless, hopeless and helpless alcoholic or addict, descending into absolute chaos and losing absolutely everything dear to them. Using what we consider to be a RATS approach to maintaining sobriety can turn their life around! We hope that we have distilled this into concepts and terms that pretty well anyone can understand.

Preface

Whilst the focus of this document primarily revolves around substance misuse, its background theoretical and practical bases are so often paralleled in other behavioural areas under the umbrella of mental health. Gambling, Eating Disorders and Obsessive-Compulsive Disorder are examples that show similar traits and can perhaps be managed in a similar fashion.

Starting with some discussion about what 'addictive behaviour' is and its potentially destructive effects, the focus turns to a simplified consideration about how it might begin in chemical terms (the substance), biological and psychological/emotional terms (the individual factors). Then there are the public attitudes towards alcoholics and addicts at the social level which add another dimension. Obviously, these 'levels' do not have clear boundaries between them and do overlap. The causes of our behaviour do not fall clearly into any one of these three and might reflect variable interactions for each one of us. We are all individuals and should be treated as such in seeking our own unique pathway in recovery.

This 'semi-scientific background' is followed by an outline of treatment methods in both medical and social contexts, their advantages and disadvantages, success rates and progresses to the life-long part of permanent abstinence. It is in this latter context that peer support within the community seems to be so vital and is probably the 'raison d'être' of organisations such as AA, NA, CA, GA and numerous other recovery-focused groups around the world, regardless of how they work. Mankind is, after all, a social animal.

In the UK at present, the transition from emergency hospital admission, through a treatment programme, to community-based peer support is not seamless. There are too many opportunities to lose momentum once the process has started and this so often leads to catastrophic relapse into the old behaviour. Of course, at all stages, the sufferer must actually want to recover and not just be paying lip-service to please family and others.

This latter point is absolutely central to success in recovery - you have to do it for yourself and no-one else. This makes it sound a very selfish process – it is! As you achieve your goal(s), the benefits for those around you will come automatically, even if it is in a new life because you have lost your old one. A sad fact that is so often true.

Habit, Compulsive Behaviour, Addiction or Dependency?

These are words that we hear so often in relation to any form of repetitive behaviour, good or bad, chemical or non-chemical. Is it useful to make any distinctions, or are they variations of a theme? The one thing that they all have in common is that it is damned hard to stop doing whatever it is! It somehow moves beyond that over-simplistic, often sanctimonious and pious view that "All it takes is willpower". Think of the willpower and thought that is required for a drug addict to score illegal drugs regularly and it creates a different context. OK, maybe it is misdirected, but it is still willpower! If only that willpower could be re-directed, what else might we be capable of excelling at?

Some habits are completely harmless, although they may be embarrassing for the sufferer and irritating to others. Picking your nose, for instance, doesn't really do any harm to anybody. On the other hand, is it symptomatic of some need for a 'comforter' in times of uncertainty, when there is no longer a dummy to suck on? Is it different to thumb sucking?

Maybe a habit becomes compulsive behaviour when it becomes constant and almost a ritual and becomes an addiction when we believe we cannot function normally without it. It becomes a true dependency when we really cannot function normally without it and it then starts to have a negative impact on your own life and the lives of others. Many addictions are probably purely psychological in their dependency whilst others, such as that to alcohol, also exhibit physiological dependency. In alcohol dependency, its physiological aspect makes sudden cessation of drinking hazardous and potentially fatal. In this case, a controlled detoxification/reduction is highly desirable. Many do try sudden cessation without detox medication and get away with it, but maybe it is not to be recommended.

The 'however' part to all of this is the transition from 'normal' behaviour, through the habit phase and onto full-blown dependency. In the case of alcohol, is wanting one or two units every day dependency, even though it is within weekly recommendations? Then there is the binge drinker, who may go for weeks or months without a drink and then have variable periods of absolutely chaotic drinking, before returning to abstinence. Similar issues are also seen in drug use. So called 'recreational' use is probably harmless but, again, it can so easily move onto dependency. Throw a mix of alcohol and a variety of drugs into the recipe and we are in different territory – or are we? We are still using substances to alter something within our 'psyche', whatever cocktail we use.

In a modern context, where does the so-called 'addiction' to computer games and smart phones fit in? It seems to fall under the heading of compulsive behaviour, particularly for the younger generation, but does it do any harm? Certainly, there is an increase in social isolation, with people hiding away and communicating electronically, rather than face to face. Following on from this, there may be a reduction in social skills that could have an influence on the quality of life, for instance in job interviews. Computer games can bring with them an apparent 'normalisation' of violence with so many of them having war-based themes. Could this lead to some vulnerable people acting out those games in real life? Only time will tell!

Dependencies seem to be filling some kind of void within ourselves, but they have 'taken control' over our behaviour and end up creating further voids and chaos. Substance misuse is, perhaps, the one that attracts most attention, probably because it creates the most widespread and visible personal and social catastrophe. People cause chaos, become physically and mentally ill or die as a direct result. Or they can get into recovery and improve their lives! Perhaps tragically, this is so often a new life because they have destroyed their old one and are forced to start again. Unfortunately, memories of that old life do not go away but have to be learned from, yet kept in the past. That pain and guilt about the past can be destructive in the new life but must serve as a valuable lesson. A return to that life is unthinkable and it may be only one drink or hit away. There is a general consensus that a return to 'normal' or 'recreational' use should not be considered. The experience of so many is that attempts to try that course of action invariably lead to disaster and abstinence is by far the best goal. Surely, if you have to control your drinking habits then you have a problem?

A few words of caution might be useful here, concerning the terms "alcoholic" and "junky". Both terms carry social stigma and often get ignored in discussion of our own behaviour, leading to that most dreaded word in this game – DENIAL!

You will have heard things like "I do drink (use) a lot, but I'm not an alcoholic (addict)". Just add the word YET to that sentence. Another might be "I would cut down, BUT it makes me feel better and I can't at the moment".

Those two three lettered words are arguably the most powerful blocks to doing anything about the problem. Just because your addiction to whatever hasn't led to you sleeping on the streets, or waking up in hospital for the umpteenth time, it DOES NOT mean that you can consider yourself to be free from those labels. Furthermore, your blood tests might show up as "normal" at that time, but it DOES NOT mean there is no sub-clinical damage that can tip-over to a danger point later in life if you do not change your behaviour. It IS NOT a green-light to continue that lifestyle with impunity.

If you are questioning your usage in any way it is time for some serious honesty, with yourself.

Recreational use of substances is viewed by many as socially acceptable and a normal part of life, until that usage gets out of control and causes chaos. Society seems to take a very dim view of people who fall foul of addictive behaviour, somewhat different to the view on other mental health issues such as depression or anxiety. The further down that substance misuse road that you get, the more of an outcast you become. You are perceived as weak-willed and useless and nothing could be further from the truth. The willpower required to get that drink or fix and keep the habit going is tremendous! Is that just misdirected willpower that can be easily turned around? The simple answer to that is a very bold and loud "NO". It is damned hard to redirect that willpower, unless the proverbial penny drops in your own brain. The man or woman who finally identifies exactly where that penny is in your brain, and how to deal with the 'switch' that needs to be 'repaired' in order to break that craving, will be a very deserving Nobel Prize winner!

The Neuroscience

This is very complicated, involving various brain regions, but an oversimplified model can help anyone to get a grasp of what seems to be going on with any repetitive behaviour that gives some kind of 'reward'. There is then the subsequent 'battle' that happens between instinct and intellect that we have all experienced in active addiction. We know that what we are doing is wrong on an intellectual level, but find our conscious selves helpless in telling the so-called pleasure centre(s) of the brain to stop driving us to do it.

Unfortunately, the concept of centres in the brain can be misleading since we are often dealing with different anatomical regions that interact to form functional 'centres', rather than truly discrete anatomical regions. Add to that the observation that centres inter-communicate and we are in trouble! Apologies to the neuroscientists for what is about to follow; we know that it is inaccurate through over-simplification, but here goes!

In our defence, in groups we have heard 'experts' talking about the amygdala, the hippocampus and nucleus accumbens in trying to explain what is going on. We have also watched 'the lights go out' in people around the room as they have simply not understood a word! We might as well be talking about an armadillo, hippopotamus and nuclear bomb. We do sometimes wonder just who these experts are trying to impress when addressing a lay audience

The central nervous system comprises the brain and spinal cord, very much the control centres that keep us alive. For simplicity, we will start by thinking of the brain in terms of higher centres, midbrain and brainstem, with the spinal cord running down the spinal column to connect with our peripheral tissues. These have a myriad of nerve networks that deal with our everyday life:

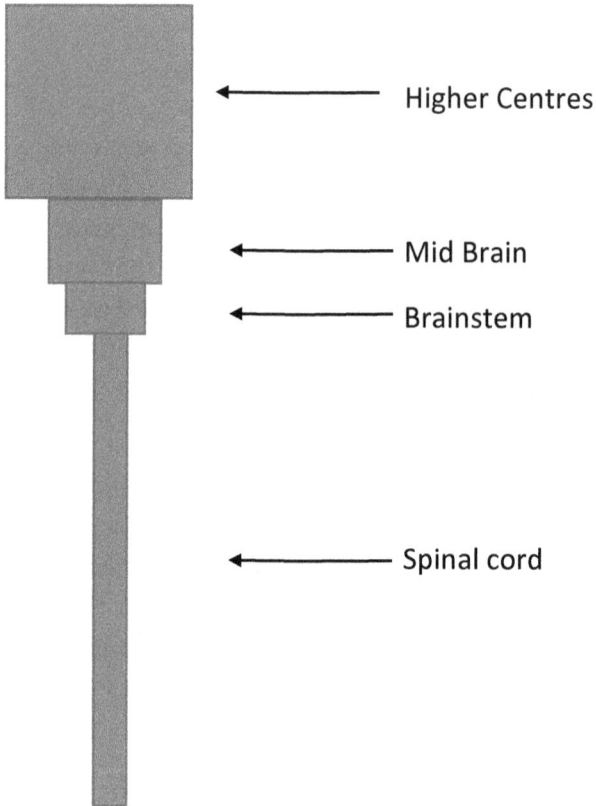

We share this basic structure with all other vertebrate mammals, but it is the higher brain that differentiates us humans. We think, we analyse, feel complex emotions and can screw ourselves up completely as a result! The midbrain, brainstem and spinal cord are concerned more with keeping us alive at an 'automatic' level, although this can often be modified by input from the higher centres.

We need little more knowledge of the brain than this to grasp a basic understanding of what might be going on in addiction. Yes, the neuroscientists are constantly learning more of the fine detail and the roles of various sub-sectors of the brain, but we have no need to know about the amygdalae, the dorso-lateral region of the neo-cortex or the hippocampus. There is a serious risk of jargonising and over-complicating the basics that we as addicts need to understand.

No-one knows exactly how many nerve cells there are in the human brain, but estimates run at about 86 billion. It is the brain that is the focus of our interest in addictive behaviour. Consequences in the spinal cord or peripheral nerves tend to be longer term effects of assaulting the body with foreign substances, not a cause of the problem. With such a vast number of cells in the brain, with all sorts of interconnections, the scope for things going wrong can only be imagined!

Of great significance in addiction is the way in which individual cells connect with each other to transmit electrical signals across the tiny gaps between cells (the synapses). This is achieved using chemical release by one cell which then acts on the next cell to generate its own electrical activity. These chemicals are collectively called neurotransmitters, of which there is a considerable variety

Some examples you may have heard of: acetylcholine, noradrenaline, serotonin (5-hydroxytryptamine), dopamine, tyramine, phenylethylamine and so the list goes on and on. They occur in different regions of the nervous system, but fulfil the same role as local chemical messengers between nerve cells. The cell on the receiving end of the signal has very specific receptors for the chemical in question. An important concept here is that all these chemicals, and similar ones, occur naturally in the biological world, both plant and animal. Even if not chemically identical, they may be close enough in their molecular structure to stimulate those receptors and, hey presto, we have plant-based drugs! Whoopee, or not? Many have sound therapeutic uses but can also be abused. A flip side to the coin is to "block" the chemical messenger in some way so that it has a reduced effect and such substances are also abundant in nature and they too often have valuable therapeutic use, or can be abused.

We now have a very complicated picture of millions of cells being regulated by a host of different chemicals alongside a range of other chemicals that may "fool" the nervous system into believing that it is controlling itself. Such a mind-blowing scenario probably explains why we know relatively little about what makes our brains tick!

A further dimension to consider concerns what goes on inside the brain cells. There is an unimaginable array of chemical reactions, both breaking down and making different substances that might act as internal messengers or regulators and be of relevance to the addictive state.

Of course, we should also not forget the consequences of substance misuse for the brain itself as its function changes in response to both short and long-term consumption, in terms of temporary changes and permanent damage. Apart from immediate death in response to massive overdose, examples of such effects include short term drunkenness, paranoia with cannabis and Wernicke-Korsakoff Syndrome as the permanent damage of chronic alcoholism.

Chemical Addiction

So how does all this fit into our crazy world of being dependent on some chemical substance that we buy from an off-licence, pharmacy or some street dealer? What is about to follow is a very oversimplified model of what might be going on inside our heads, for which we must apologise to the scientific purists.

Start out by thinking about eating food and stopping to eat – maybe when we are full, or not! There is no way in which our intermittent eating pattern matches closely the use of nutrients by the body from moment to moment. This means that something much cleverer than the following level of description is actually involved, but here goes.

Hunger is a biological drive to eat and when the control system thinks we have had enough food, satiety switches this drive off. This is similar to a simple room thermostat turning the heating on and off and would provide some sort of rather imprecise control, but it could work. Now, we need to add appetite into the recipe; this is a desire to eat a certain type of food, for instance chocolate. Chocolate is very pleasurable and this can override the satiety that is trying to stop us eating. Conversely, coal is not appetising and we would soon spit it out; it is also of no nutritional value, unlike the chocolate. Put simply, chocolate stimulates a pleasure-based reflex to continue eating it and we can become addicted to it. The end result of this can be damage to teeth and obesity in the short term and death through heart disease in the long term. In other words it damages our bodies! Sounding familiar?

Pleasure centre(s) in the brain are well recognised and it is not difficult to understand how taking substances such as alcohol or other drugs can stimulate them. The obvious question is why this pleasure response doesn't switch off and we simply stop using whatever it is before it becomes problematic? He or she who can answer that question also deserves a Nobel Prize! The neuroscientists have moved a long way towards understanding the cellular level of addiction, but it has yet to yield answers that drug and alcohol therapists can use reliably and across the board. Yes, something that is believed to act as a kind of switch at the cellular level has been identified, but translating that through to therapy at the thinking human being level seems a long way off!

A useful way to think of this switch might be to liken it to a spring-loaded door. Taking the pleasurable substance forces the door open, but then the spring closes it again and you stop taking the substance. Repeated use, however, weakens that spring and eventually it breaks, leaving the door flapping and the substance can flood in. Allied to that, with repeated use, it also takes more of the substance to give the same effect at the conscious level. At this point the control system has been hijacked and the door cannot close automatically. You are well and truly addicted and being controlled by the substance.

Nature being what it is, it has provided an alternative means for closing this door, using the higher brain. We have to learn ways of closing that door using conscious means and, through repetition, condition the higher brain to keep that door closed. Unfortunately, we are trying to use a conscious mind that might be completely screwed up, perhaps through emotional distresses or damage that we have caused through the addiction itself, never mind that caused before you started using any substance.

In this context, we need to reconsider that concept of "pleasure" to embrace the fact that our use of a substance might be providing some inner relief from deep seated emotional distress. Such distress might go as far back in the mists of time to your early years and is out of conscious memory with no obvious link to your problem. Equally, it might be related to something more recent and you are 'using' to 'help you through it' and then can't stop. Maybe this is a distorted take on the concept but it makes some sense and helps to explain why we start to overuse substances in the first place. The difficulty, as always, is that when we stop taking the substance, the problem and feelings are still there, so we have to keep using. What a "Catch 22" situation to be in!

Approaches to Therapy

It might be fair to say that there are as many approaches to recovery as there are addicts who have recovered. They range from those who simply made a decision one day that they should stop using and did so successfully for the rest of their lives, through to those who require numerous attempts at rehab and lifelong support, usually as part of groups. Then there are those who give up trying and may have a long, slow, painful and early death. If at first you don't succeed ...... you know the rest! Please give up any ideas you might have of finding out how or why you fell-foul of the addiction curse. It is impossible, so you must focus whole-heartedly on your recovery.

Regardless of any scientific and spiritual merit, or otherwise, probably the most widely known approach is the Alcoholics Anonymous Twelve Step programme developed in the USA during the 1930s. This has been adopted and adapted to suit other addictions such as Narcotics Anonymous, Cocaine Anonymous and Gamblers Anonymous. It now has a history of over 80 years and is still going strong, providing support for the rest of a person's life if they feel that they need it. This is in stark contrast to residential or community-based rehabilitation services that abandon their clients when they have completed their programme.

The "non-fellowship" programmes may work with the 12 Step Programme or other theoretical orientations, such as Cognitive Behavioural Therapy (CBT) or Acceptance and Commitment Therapy (ACT). Whichever approach is used, the real aim is to stop using the substance and stay stopped. Many say that stopping is the easy part and staying stopped is the hard part (for the rest of your life?). Of course, there are some individuals, probably a minority, who are able to return to "social or controlled use" of the substance. Unfortunately, the long-term success rate of any approach is virtually impossible to measure. There are always people who start a programme and then give up only to disappear under the radar and any potential data is lost. We have no idea about their fates, but can probably hazard a very good guess – continued use and early death!

Intuitively, it is probably a fair guess that less than 10% of people who start any programme actually achieve sustained recovery lasting years. Realistically, data collection and validation is nigh-on impossible. Even the fellowships do not keep a register of attendance at meetings; they are, after all, anonymous and consequently there are no records of individuals and/or sobriety duration.

Nevertheless, the 12 Step programme has a long-standing record and provides a really useful starting point for piecing together the key stages of any recovery programme. At this point, it is worth remembering that old adage "If at first you don't succeed, try, try and try again". So many people don't succeed at the first attempt and it is better to think of yourself as a serial trier rather than a serial relapser. It can be a real revolving door of relapse and success, each phase being of unpredictable duration.

The Twelve Steps

1) We admitted we were powerless over alcohol - that our lives had become unmanageable.

2) Came to believe that a Power greater than ourselves could restore us to sanity.

3) Made a decision to turn our will and our lives over to the care of God as we understood Him.

4) Made a searching and fearless moral inventory of ourselves.

5) Admitted to God, to ourselves and to another human being the exact nature of our wrongs.

6) Were entirely ready to have God remove all these defects of character.

7) Humbly asked Him to remove our shortcomings.

8) Made a list of all persons we had harmed, and became willing to make amends to them all.

9) Made direct amends to such people wherever possible, except when to do so would injure them or others.

10) Continued to take personal inventory and when we were wrong promptly admitted it.

11) Sought through prayer and meditation to improve our conscious contact with God as we understood Him, praying only for knowledge of His will for us and the power to carry that out.

12) Having had a spiritual awakening as the result of these steps, we tried to carry this message to alcoholics and to practice these principles in all our affairs.

This is probably the most widely used approach to dealing with substance misuse and has a history spanning many decades, but it can seem very daunting. It is an ongoing process that cannot be completed in one week, or one month, but aims to change your life in a gradual, permanent way. It needs ongoing commitment for the rest of your existence to maintain your sobriety. Having said that, other approaches to therapy often attempt to do the same thing(s).

Many people, however, have trouble with the programme for a variety of reasons which are often difficult to pin down. Some of the most obvious are:

- Its aim is total abstinence. Many feel that they would like to return to 'normal' social drinking and do not wish to abstain completely. Experience shows, however, that this applies to only a small proportion of people since the probability of serious relapse is much greater if you are still dabbling.

- It has a strong element of religious and spiritual belief and development, with little or no obvious scientific basis. This is reinforced by the simple fact that meetings often take place in church halls and some perceive it as some kind of cult. This makes commitment by atheists or agnostics more of a challenge.

- Making a list of all the people harmed seems almost impossible if everyone you have harmed or offended is to be included, never mind the obvious practical difficulties in 'making amends' to them. Attempts to make amends could in themselves be met with a variety of responses and could be counter-productive; they have nothing to do with being 'forgiven' or any other helpful response. Dealing with your own guilt is a tough one.

- It relies on group work and interaction, many believing that they should be able to succeed without that kind of support. Equally, a lot of people simply hate the idea of sharing in a group, perhaps preferring a one-to-one approach. This can be achieved by the use of a sponsor from the Fellowship, but it does narrow down the range of lived experience that you are exposed to.

- On the face of it, it requires a lifelong commitment to attending meetings. A stark reality here is that those people with 20 years under their belt have indeed usually kept their meetings up. Those that do not are not tracked and there is no record of their success or failure. Take your pick!

All in all, this is a very daunting prospect that leaves many feeling cold. Of course, over the decades since this programme came to fruition, there have been real developments in the biological and psychological understanding of addiction and there are newer approaches, such as CBT, ACT and others. Whilst these might sometimes seem to be polar opposites of the 12-Step approach, there are similarities, even if they seem to be mirror images.

That is, to some extent, the 12-Step programme might be seen as "Change your behaviour with this programme and your thinking will follow" whilst CBT tries to "Change your thinking and your behaviour will follow". Get the point? A striking difference between the two is in the aftercare once you have made significant progress. This also applies to people undergoing residential rehabilitation by any programme. You leave the rehab and you are left to fend for yourself. Complete an (expensive?) CBT programme of therapy and you are again on your own when it's finished.

Take a scenario where you have had numerous emergency hospital admissions, are detoxed each time and at last sent to a funded residential rehab for 3 months. Whatever the programme followed in the rehab, this has cost the state, or you, megabucks and you are discharged with nowhere to go for ongoing support. At least with the 12-Step programme, you have somewhere to go for support each day or each week. In all honesty, some kind of ongoing support is invaluable for keeping you on the straight and narrow and many services will steer you towards the 12-Step Fellowships.

In various parts of the UK, and the rest of the world, there are now peer support groups/communities springing up that have no core therapeutic philosophy. They are there to provide that on-going support that seems to be so valuable, maybe meeting once a week and/or offering specific activities such as art. They may appear to be little more than social/discussion groups with recovery as an underlying theme. They do, however, seem to work and often provide a broader experience, simply because they are not influenced by any particular doctrine. We all ended up in the mire by different routes and there are as many different pathways of getting out of it!

We like to think of the whole scenario as resembling a tree. The roots (routes?) are the bits in the earth (mire), all coming together in the trunk (starting recovery process) from different directions and developing through different branches and twigs until we become the leaves. Hopefully, we are on an evergreen tree and don't drop off in the autumn! We all got out of the darkness and into the daylight in different ways.

Core Requirements of Recovery

So, what exactly seem to be the key themes running through any successful approach to therapy? It is worthwhile casting an eye over those 12-Steps and trying to pull out key features that might help you to overcome the hurdles they seem to present you with. We could almost whittle this down to a 'Fewer-Step Programme' and maybe add some bolt-ons! Having said that, even the 12-Steps themselves do not have to be completed in a numerical order and AA members will tell you that you can adapt sequence and interpret steps to suit yourself. You might be told that your higher power could be as simple as a coffee table which, at the time, gives little faith in the programme! Point taken though, it doesn't have to be some kind of deity, it could be something more tangible, like the group itself.

The first thing we need to recognise is that there is no 'magic bullet' to fixing an alcoholic or drug addict. Yes, there are medications that can help you along the way, perhaps by suppressing craving, acting as less harmful substitutes or even making you ill if you do drink or use. These are, however, tools and not cures. We rely heavily on psychological and social support to really bring things under control.

That one word, control, is important. There is, as yet, no evidence that addictive behaviour can be cured in the true sense of the word, just the same as it is for so many other 'psychiatric' disorders. Things are brought under control using medicines and/or psycho-social interventions; the condition is not eradicated and we have to accept that. The thing that needs to be eradicated from your mind is any kind of euphoric/romantic memory of happy times when you were able to indulge sensibly; those days are over.

The stuff has wrecked your life in some way and that is what you must remember!

That leads us nicely into piecing together the core requirements of treatment. Whist these are numbered, it does not imply for one minute that there is a particular sequence, perhaps with the exception of number 1! Even so, we often need to revisit this at intervals if we are getting over-confident about our recovery and the same is true of the other numbers. The whole thing is a dynamic and iterative process.

1) Admit defeat: The stuff has beaten you; it controls you and not you control it. It has wrecked your life in some way; you have hit rock-bottom. This varies a lot from the relatively minor, such as it ended your marriage, through to the disastrous where you add

career, home, family, car and dog to the list and are living on the streets as drunk/stoned as a skunk.

2) Want to change: Really, this is a natural follow on to the above, but it is absolutely essential. You have to want if for yourself and no-one else. Not the wife/husband and/or kids, but for yourself. You also have to be ready to commit to your recovery wholeheartedly and this might take a relapse or few before you get there.

3) Ask for help: Start with human beings, such as your doctor, nurse, social worker, local treatment service, local fellowship groups, a rehabilitation centre or even a bookshop/library. The collective human experience is so important but some kind of medical input is valuable in the very early days when you might be at risk of some withdrawal catastrophe, or you are unaware of an existing pathological condition.

4) Listen: This is essential whether you are in one-to-one therapy or partaking in group work. So often, you are with people who have their own experience of the condition and recovery and may have a lot of sober time under their belt. You almost certainly will not feel comfortable with a lot of what you hear but some of it will strike a real chord with you. If it worked for them it might work for you, but no-one is telling you exactly what to do. You build your own programme on a pick and mix basis.

5) Look within: This sort of equates with steps 4, 8, 9 and 10 of the 12-Step Programme but also allies with what CBT and ACT aim to do. That is to look at your thinking and habits, change them as necessary and then your overall behaviour will change. The bits in the 12-Step approach about making a list of people you have harmed and making amends where possible may well be frankly impossible, but you really do need to acknowledge the harm and chaos that you have caused. This can be approached by sharing it with other(s) in one-to-one or group work. Just vocalising it can work wonders. An alternative might be to write it down as a life history, or in poetry;

you can always subsequently burn all that 'garbage' as a symbolic 'letting-go'.

6) Be patient: It so often took many years to get into the mess you are in and you will not get out of it overnight. Try not to make other life changing decisions without a fair chunk of sober time under your own belt. There is no hard and fast guideline on how long this should be, but it is probably at the very least 6 months – or preferably longer. You are not yet in a position to go out and save the world from addiction.

7) Keep it up: Don't get cocky and feel that you have got it sorted. The problem doesn't disappear, it just goes into hiding waiting for you to drop your guard and relapse. Remember, addiction is a very patient condition and it might be several years before it bites you on the backside again. Keeping up with your support network is the most useful way of doing this part - staying sober. Some say that giving up is easy and it is staying clean that is the really hard part.

Please remember that these are not arranged in any particular sequence, they are merely suggestions to help you find your own way forward. Everyone got in to similar shades of mess but by very different routes and maybe different end-points. It is not compulsory to end up as a homeless vagrant to see the light! Equally, everyone can climb out of the pit using different strategies that suit them.

Some of these practical strategies to help prevent relapse can be learned from people with more time and experience under their belt. Others you will be introduced to as part of a programme organised by your local community-based treatment service. It is not too difficult to find your local service through health professionals or online and they are well worth a try.

Remember, relapse is not a failure but is remarkably common, with three relapses being a bit of a rule of thumb before you really get the hang of it. Each relapse serves as a reminder and provides an opportunity to re-examine things and try to identify where it went wrong. They do serve as a stark reminder about the seriousness of your condition and the need to focus on your recovery. The main thing is not to overthink things but to pick yourself up, dust yourself down, get back on your bike and keep pedalling. It is all part of becoming well and truly ready to commit whole-heartedly to your recovery. A friend in sustained recovery from addiction and mental health issues puts it quite well as:

"If you stay in your head, you're as good as dead; listen to your heart and make a start".

Whatever approach is used in therapy, please remember that long term success rates are nigh on impossible to measure but seem to be very low. Nevertheless, it is probably worth hanging on to the observation that people with sustained recovery have generally kept up with some kind of support network. Perhaps it is not compulsory that this involves fellows in recovery, but these are the people who have real experience of your struggles and understand you best. Having said that, if you can find non-addicts who can empathise with you then that might also be useful. These may be people who live with other mental health issues such as anxiety or depression or maybe other apparently more serious conditions. You would be surprised just how much common ground you can share.

It might also help you to realise that yours is a condition in which your choices alone are the real key to success. Albeit very hard to do, you can choose not to use the substance(s)! After all, abandoning these chemicals is the key to success, rather than taking others prescribed by a doctor. If you suffer from other conditions, such as bipolar disorder or autistic spectrum, drug treatment might be the best or only way of managing your condition. Even in those cases, peer support can be an extremely useful adjunct to drug therapy.

Cockney Intro

Well, here we are again after some more soul bearing poetry we have decided to call upon our dear friend the crazy cockney. These visits have provided us, and hopefully you, with a good laugh after the seriousness of the initial poems and the battles so many of us face daily. As we take one last stroll on the cobbles, we want to thank you for joining us on this journey and we hope it has been of some support and help.

A Cockney on the Cobbles III

'Allo mush, ain't seen you for donkeys, 'ow's life bin treetin yer!

'Ow long yer got mate? It's bin a rite bleedin rolla coasta. Let's go getta Rosie and I'll tell yer all about it.

OK, there's a greasy spoon round the corner

Grab a pew, open yer King Lears and lissen. Life finally caught up wiv me. It wasn't just the grog, I got 'eavy into the Persians as well. You name it, green, white, 'orse, I tried the bleedin' lot and then lost the plot. 'Er indoors told me to foxtrot, drifted into a den and met some aver Bacardis. One of 'em, the General, ended up pushin' up daisies after an 'eavy binge. Fit young feller 'e woz till 'e dropped brahn bread in front of me. I 'ad to go apple bobbin' to get me supplies and got caught red 'anded. I woz 'alf inchin' a custard but forgot the remote and went back in. Came out to a street full of plod and blues and tried to leg it. One rozzer tugged me collar so I stuck the nut in and dahn we both went. The beak gave me a five stretch but I got aht in three. That bit of porridge switched a lite on in me loaf thanks to me cell mate. 'E woz a real veteran of the game, blags, bombs and running toms, 'e made a real career of it. When the Scotch Mist cleared, 'e realised he was just bein' a berk and figured that 'e needed to jack it all in. We'd often rabbit about bein' away from it all and that there must be more to life. 'E woz such a veteran that 'e still 'as some years but I got aht to an 'ostel. Trouble and tin lids are long gone and it is just me in that little room. Lesson learned and I am now clean and as a judge. Keep me napper dahn and "Carry on Sergeant".

Good on yer me ole China, stay safe and I'll see yer dahn the frog sometime.

And Finally

Whatever your issues, we wish you the best of luck in your therapy. We have had a degree of success in our apparently *very* different conditions and have found great value in working together, forming a highly valued (if most unlikely) friendship and support bubble. Nevertheless, we still use our wider support network(s) that focus more on our own conditions.

Stay safe, stay positive and keep right on to the end of the road.

Life will get better!

And they all lived happily ever after...........

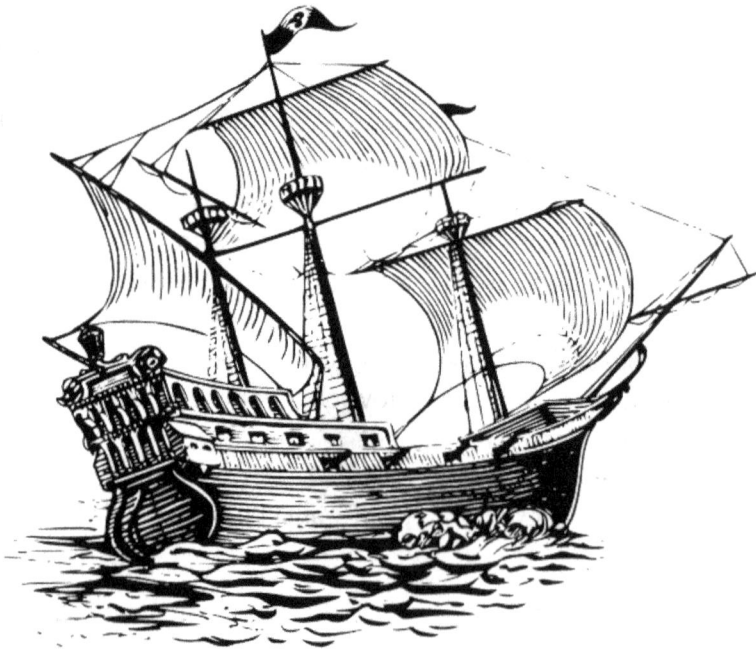

www.ingramcontent.com/pod-product-compliance
Lightning Source LLC
Chambersburg PA
CBHW060119050426
42448CB00010B/1934